Embryology and Anomalies
of the Facial Nerve
and Their Surgical Implications

Embryology and Anomalies of the Facial Nerve and Their Surgical Implications

Robert Thayer Sataloff, MD, DMA

Professor of Otolaryngology
Thomas Jefferson University
Philadelphia, PA

Illustrated by:
Zaven Jabourian, MD
Assistant Professor of Otolaryngology
Thomas Jefferson University
Philadelphia, PA

RAVEN PRESS ✦ NEW YORK

Raven Press, Ltd., 1185 Avenue of the Americas, New York, New York 10036

Made in the United States of America

Library of Congress Cataloging-in-Publication Data

Sataloff, Robert Thayer.
    Embryology of the facial nerve / Robert Thayer Sataloff ; illustrated by Zaven Jabourian.
        p.   cm.
    ISBN 0-88167-728-0
    1. Facial nerve—Growth. I. Title.
    [DNLM: 1. Facial Nerve—abnormalities. 2. Facial Nerve—
embryology. WL 330 S253e]
    QM471.S33   1990
    611.6'40183—dc20
    DNLM/DLC
    for Library of Congress   90-9016
                                             CIP

The material contained in this volume was submitted as previously unpublished material, except in the instances in which credit has been given to the source from which some of the illustrative material was derived.

Great care has been taken to maintain the accuracy of the information contained in the volume. However, neither Raven Press nor the editors can be held responsible for errors or for any consequences arising from the use of the information contained herein.

Materials appearing in this book prepared by individuals as part of their official duties as U.S. Government employees are not covered by the above-mentioned copyright.

9 8 7 6 5 4 3 2 1

To my father, partner, and best friend
Joseph Sataloff, MD, DSC,
whose guidance and inspiration are largely responsible
for any successes I have enjoyed in my profession

Preface

This book is the result of more than ten years of inquiry. It began when I was a resident in the Department of Otorhinolaryngology at the University of Michigan. The teaching at that time suggested that the location of the facial nerve in congenitally malformed ears was unknown. This produced uncertainty and fear in the otologic surgeon. In fact, many otolaryngologists were opposed to corrective surgery for hearing improvement especially in patients with unilateral malformations, believing that the risk of facial paralysis was greater than the potential gain. It seemed to me that if one understood the embryology of the facial nerve, it would be possible to make a reasonably accurate prediction of facial nerve position in most cases. However, when I went to the library to look up facial nerve embryology and correlate it with embryology of the ear, I found the literature review almost more challenging than the surgery itself.

Some of this book is based on a study that was undertaken to help solve the practical clinical problem of facial nerve localization in surgical candidates with congenitally malformed ears. This study won the Edmund Prince Fowler Award for basic research, presented by the American Rhinological, Laryngological and Otological (Triological) Society in 1989. The information in this book will prove convenient and practical for otologic surgeons and students of otologic embryology and will facilitate review of this fascinating subject.

Acknowledgments

I am deeply indebted to many people for assistance in the preparation of this book. First, my deepest appreciation goes to my father, Joseph Sataloff, who inspired me to enter otolaryngology and advised me to train at the University of Michigan, and who has continued to share his wisdom with me throughout our years in practice together. The academic and clinical training I received from Walter P. Work, Charles J. Krause, Malcolm D. Graham, and others in Ann Arbor has been invaluable; as was my exposure in Los Angeles with Bill and Howard House and their associates. I am indebted to all of my mentors for helping prepare me to write this text. This work was also aided immeasurably by Merle Lawrence, Ph.D., who was kind enough to permit me to study his collection of embryology slides. I am also indebted to Kyle Rarey, Ph.D. for making Dr. Lawrence's slide collection available to me again recently for reassessment and for his invaluable assistance in reviewing histologic materials. It is impossible to thank adequately my friend and colleague Zaven Jabourian, M.D. During his first and second years in practice as an otolaryngologist, he generously donated his time, talent, and friendship to render the illustrations in this book. They are superb, and the fact that they were drawn by an otolaryngologist made the process immeasurably easier. A very special debt of gratitude goes to Mary Hawkshaw, R.N., B.S.N., my nurse, editorial assistant, and patient friend, who devoted almost as many hours to this manuscript and its photographs as I did. Without her dedicated and expert assistance, preparation of this book probably would have taken another year or two. I also express my gratitude to Helen Caputo, who retyped the manuscript more times than either of us can count, and to Kathy Mayer for her assistance in labeling the illustrations. Finally, I express deep appreciation to my understanding and tolerant wife, Dahlia Sataloff, M.D., who put up with innumerable ruined evenings, weekends, vacations, and summer trips while I was engrossed in completing this project.

I am indebted to the Triological Society and the Laryngoscope for permission to republish materials from my article "Embryology of the Facial Nerve and Its Clinical Applications," including portions of the text and Table 2, and Figures 18, 21, 24, 31, 33, 40–44, 47, 49–53, 56–58, 60, 62–65.

Contents

Embryology and Anomalies of the Facial Nerve and Their Surgical Implications

1

Introduction

The hazards of surgery upon congenitally malformed ears are well recognized and stressed in otolaryngologic training programs. Special caution is advised because the surgeon cannot depend upon anatomic landmarks or their customary relationships to each other. Concern about the facial nerve is generally emphasized because in congenitally malformed ears, allegedly, "you never know where you are going to find it." This widely promulgated notion is useful for prompting appropriate caution in the otologic surgeon and a thorough preoperative discussion of potential complications with the patient. But when operating on a malformed ear, it should be possible for the surgeon to predict with reasonable accuracy the course of the facial nerve. Radiologic studies including computed tomography are helpful in many cases, but structural anomalies and absence of the fallopian canal may render them insufficient in some patients.

It seemed logical that if one understood the development of the facial nerve and its changes in position during fetal growth, then one should be able to predict its position at a specific point in development. It also seemed likely that if the facial nerve were abnormal, arrest of facial nerve development in the temporal bone would generally occur at the same time as developmental arrest of other structures in a malformed ear. Malformations of the external ear are easy to observe visually, and malformations of the middle ear and inner ear can generally be defined well by radiologic imaging. Therefore, a study was designed not only to describe the embryology of the facial nerve, but also to correlate its development sequentially with the growth of the ear. Although embryology of the ear has been described well, it is surprising that nearly all of the literature discusses embryology of the outer ear, middle ear, and inner ear separately. Consequently, no source was found prior to 1986 to which a surgeon could turn to learn quickly the developmental state of all three divisions of the ear at a given point in time. For example, if one identified an auricular anomaly as occurring at 16 weeks, there was no comprehensive article or book that described the development of the ossicles, the middle ear space, and the cochlea at 16 weeks without laborious review of the embryologic development of each of these structures individually. Moreover, there is virtually no literature prior to 1986 that describes facial nerve development temporally in conjunction with developing ear structures.

Embryology of the facial nerve is as fascinating as it is complex. Its peculiar course in the human adult, intimate relationship with otologic structures encountered routinely by surgeons, and its functional importance have inspired studies of facial nerve development for more than a century. Although most of these articles present only a partial description of facial nerve development, a few recent investigators have provided a much more complete description of facial nerve embryology.

In addition to providing information on embryology of the facial nerve and its clinical applications, this book includes chapters on anomalies of the facial nerve. It is hoped that these chapters prove valuable to the clinician concerned with diagnosis and treatment of facial nerve disorders.

2

Embryology of the Facial Nerve

The comprehensive analysis of the development of the facial nerve presented here was developed from several sources. It represents a synthesis of selected articles on facial nerve embryology (1–56), information available in literature not specifically involved with the facial nerve but containing illustrations of embryos in which the facial nerve is pictured (57–60), studies of histologic sections of human fetuses from Dr. Merle Lawrence's collection at the University of Michigan, Ann Arbor, Michigan, and dissection of fetal heads. Dissection of eight fetal heads under the fertilization age of 16 weeks provided very little useful information. Where accurate observations were possible, they confirmed the findings illustrated in previous literature. It was possible to obtain only one older specimen. Although dissection of this specimen was more revealing, studies of histologic preparations provided considerably more information and are used more extensively in this book. Histologic slides are presented from 24 ears of 19 specimens ranging from ten weeks fertilization age to seven days following full-term delivery. They were selected from approximately 2,200 histologic sections reviewed. The descriptions and drawings of facial nerve embryology presented represent a composite of information gleaned from these various published and original sources. A few particularly thorough articles have been of special importance in our understanding of facial nerve embryology (6, 7, 24, 42, 44, 47, 50, 55, 56), although information and especially drawings and photographs in the other sources were also extremely valuable. The original histologic slides

TABLE 1. *Criteria for estimating fetal age*[a]

Fertilization age	Crown-rump length	Comment
20–21 days	1.5–3.0 mm	1–3 somites, head fold, deep neural groove.
22–23 days	2.0–3.5 mm	4–12 somites, first and second pairs of branchial arches visible. Neural tube widely open. Embryo slightly curved or straight.
24–25 days	2.5–4.5 mm	13–20 somites, otic placodes and optic vesicles present. Rostral neuropore closing. Embryo curved.
26–27 days	3.0–5.0 mm	21–29 somites, caudal neuropore closed or closing. Otic pits present. Heart prominence and upper limb spuds present. Three pairs branchial arches present.
28–30 days	4.0–6.0 mm	30–35 somites, otic vesicles present. Four pairs of branchial arches lower limb buds present. Attenuated tail present.
31–32 days	5.0–7.0 mm	Optic cuffs, lens pits, and nasal pits visible. Upper limbs are paddle-shaped.
33–36 days	7.0–9.0 mm	Nasal pits prominent. Lower limbs are paddle-shaped. Hand plates and cervical sinus present.
37–40 days	8.0–11.0 mm	Auricular hillocks, the retinal pigment, and footplates present.
41–43 days	11.0–14.0 mm	Auricular hillocks mark the future shape of auricle. Finger rays appear. Trunk begins to straighten.
44–46 days	13.0–17.0 mm	Eyelids forming. Notches between finger rays. Toe rays and nipples appear. Elbows visible.
47–48 days	16.0–18.0 mm	Trunk elongating. Limbs extend. Midgut herniation prominent.
49–51 days	18.0–22.0 mm	Fingers webbed. Upper limbs bent at elbows. Notches between toe rays.
52–53 days	22.0–24.0 mm	Fingers free. Toes webbed. Short tail present.
54–55 days	23.0–28.0 mm	Eyelids and auricles better developed. Toes no longer webbed.

TABLE 1. *Continued.*

Fertilization age	Crown-rump length	Comment
56 days	27.0–31.0 mm	Tail has disappeared. Head rounded and recognizably human. External genitalia still without recognizable sex.
9 weeks	50 mm	Head more rounded. Eyes closed or closing.
10 weeks	61 mm	Early fingernail development. Intestine in abdomen.
12 weeks	87 mm	Neck clearly recognizable. Sex recognizable externally.
14 weeks	120 mm	Head erect. Lower limbs well developed.
16 weeks	140 mm	Ears stand out from head.
18 weeks	160 mm	Early toenail development. Vernix caseosa present.
20 weeks	190 mm	Head and body hair visible.
22 weeks	210 mm	Skin wrinkled and red. Fetus viable.
24 weeks	230 mm	Fingernails present. Thin body.
26 weeks	250 mm	Eyelashes present. Eyes partially open.
28 weeks	270 mm	Eyes open. Skin slightly wrinkled. Full head of hair.
30 weeks	280 mm	Body less thin. Toenails present. Testes descending.
32 weeks	300 mm	Skin smoth and pink. Fingernails reach fingertips.
36 weeks	340 mm	Toenails reach toe tips. Lanugo hairs nearly absent. Body plump. Limbs flexed.
38 weeks	360 mm	Fingernails extend beyond fingertips. Chest and breasts prominent. Testes in scrotum or inguinal canals.

[a]Developmental stages of human embryos. Criteria for estimating fertilization age of fetuses (66–68) modified in part (68). When menstrual age is reported in the literature, fertilization age is calculated by subtracting 14 days from the menstrual age.

were stained with hematoxylin and eosin except where other stains are indicated. Various planes of section had been used that optimize visualization of the facial nerve and related structures.

In addition to describing the embryology of the facial nerve, this book correlates its development with that of related ear structures.

TABLE 2. *Summary of chronological development of the facial nerve, external ear, middle ear, and inner ear*

Week of development (fertilization age)	3	4	5
Facial nerve	Facioacoustic primordium appears and gives rise to sensory fibers of VII (Fig. 18).	Ventrally, VII approaches the epibranchial placode. Primordium splits into caudal main trunk and rostral chorda tympani (same size); chorda tympani enters mandibular arch (Fig. 19).	Nervus intermedius and geniculate ganglion visible. Greater superficial petrosal nerve appears. Twigs to posterior digastric pre-muscle mass. All cranial nerves except I and II are present. Sensory cranial nerves have visible ganglia. Orbicularis oris and levator anguli oris present (Fig. 21).
External ear		Ectoderm of first branchial groove and endoderm of first pharyngeal pouch come in contact.	
Middle ear	First and second pouches; lie lateral to primordium of oral and pharyngeal tongue. Third	Approximately 4½ weeks, second arch mesenchyme condenses to form the stapes	

		blastema. VII divides the blastema into stapes, interhyale, and laterohyale.	Wide dorsal and slender ventral part of otic vesicle appear. Between them, the endolymphatic duct and sac emerge at about where the otic vesicle separated from the superficial ectoderm. Dorsal part will become vestibular part of labyrinth. Ventral part will become cochlea. Acoustic ganglion divides into superior (vestibular) and inferior (cochlear) parts. Mesenchymal condensation is beginning of otic capsule.
Inner ear	arch enlarges and space between second arch is compressed becoming the eustachian tube. Out-pocketing of lateral end becomes middle ear space (endoderm lined first pharyngeal pouch). Neuroectoderm and ectoderm lateral to first branchial groove condense to form the otic placode. Otic placode develops in conjunction with acousticofacial ganglion, lateral to the rhombencephalon.	Otic placode invaginates to become the otic pit. Then the surface opening closes, making it the otocyst or otic vesicle. Common macula appears. Angiogenesis around the otic vesicle begins. Otic placode cells migrate through otic vesicle basement membrane to reach area where VIII ganglion will form.	

TABLE 2. *Continued.*

Week of development (fertilization age)		
6	7	8

Facial nerve		
Complete separation of VII and VIII. Discrete nervus intermedius. Greater superficial petrosal nerve joins deep petrosal to form nerve of the pterygoid canal. Geniculate ganglion is well formed and gives off a branch to the glossopharyngeal ganglion. Between weeks 6–7 (10–18 mm), superficial second arch mesenchymal lamina spreads to form occipital, cervical, mandibular, and temporal laminae. The deep lamina forms the posterior digastric complex. Submandibular ganglion develops at 6½ weeks. Although the geniculate ganglion and two intratemporal branches are well formed, there is only a suggestion of the horizontal and vertical directions that the nerve will eventually assume. At this point, it runs a fairly	Nervus intermedius is smaller than motor root. Chorda tympani and lingual nerves unite. Postauricular nerve communicates with C-2 and C-3. Peripheral VII divides into branches. Branches reach the infraorbital rim. Unbranched parotid bud is present. Posterior belly of digastric, stapedius, and stylohyoid develop. Interanastomoses of peripheral branches of VII appear by 22 mm. Branch to stapedius visible at 26 mm. Cranially coursing peripheral branches appear (zygomatic and temporal). All peripheral divisions identified by 26 mm. Communications well established with V. Buccinator, depressor anguli oris, and zygomaticus major appear. The horizontal and vertical portions of the facial nerve are now recognizable. However, they	Superficial layer of second arch mesenchyme forms infraorbital lamina and occipital platysma. Frontalis appears. Parotid approaches lower buccal, marginal mandibular, and cervical branches of VII, and second-order ductules form (27 mm). Third-order ductules form by 32 mm, and primordium enters the parotid space. By 37 mm, fourth-order ductules appear and the buccal nerve is superficial to the parotid duct. The sulcus that will become the fallopian canal appears in contact with VII, vessels, and stapedius. In the ninth week, the laterohyale fuses with the otic capsule to join Reichert's cartilage in producing the anterior wall of the fallopian canal (Fig. 36). Auricularis anterior, corrugator supercilii, occipital, and mandibular platysma appear at

			50–60 mm (9–10 weeks).
	straight course from the area of the geniculate ganglion across the region that will become the middle ear to the region of the second arch near the first groove (Figs. 23 and 24).	are still far anterior to their adult position with respect to the external auditory meatus, which is low on the head of the developing embryo (Figs. 31, 33, and 35).	

External ear	Condensation of mesoderm of first and second arches into hillocks of His.
	First arch:
	  first hillock—tragus
	  second hillock—helical crus
	  third hillock—helix
	Second arch:
	  fourth hillock—antihelix
	  fifth hillock—antitragus
	  sixth hillock—lobule and lower helix
	Concha forms from three areas of first groove *ectoderm*:
	middle part of first groove—*concha cavum*; upper part of first groove—*intertraqus incisura* (Figs. 26, 27, and 29).
		Cartilage formation (Fig. 30).	First pharygeal (ph.) groove surface ectoderm thickens and grows as solid core of epithelium toward middle ear. Auricle develops further (Fig. 39).

Middle ear	Malleus and incus appear as a single mass.	Stapes ring emerges around the stapedial artery. Lamina stapedialis (otic mesenchyme) appears to become the footplate and annular ligament. Interhyale cells aggregate as	Malleus and incus are separated and incudomalleal joint is formed. Meckel's cartilage (first arch mesoderm): head and neck of malleus, body and short process of incus.

TABLE 2. *Continued.*

Week of development (fertilization age)	6	7	8
		precursor of stapedius muscle.	Reichert's cartilage (second arch mesoderm): manubrium of malleus, long process of incus. Anterior process of malleus is from the process of folius (mesenchyme bone). At 8½ weeks, the incudostapedial joint develops, interhyale becomes the stapedial muscle and tendon. Laterohyale becomes posterior wall of middle ear and, together with the otic capsule, the pyramidal process and facial canal. The lower part of the facial canal is believed to come from Reichert's cartilage.

| Inner ear | Semicircular canals appear. Common macula has differentiated: superior (upper) part—utricular macula and cristae of superior and lateral canals; inferior (lower) part—saccular macula and cristae of posterior canal. Cartilaginous appearance of mesenchyme around otic capsule. Cochlear duct forms one turn. Endolymphatic duct appears. | Further development of basal turn of the cochlea. Depression develops between saccule and cochlear duct and constricts to form ductus reuniens. Maculae differentiate into sensory and supporting cells; cristae ampullaris form (Fig. 38). | Semicircular canals and utricle are fully formed. Sacculae and endolymphatic duct are formed. Sacculo-endolymphatic and uriculo-endolymphatic ducts form. Stria vascularis begins to develop. Two ridges of cells appear, the outer being the precursor of the organ of Corti. Precursor of otic capsule develops further as precartilage. Rugae appear in the endolymphatic sac. Vestibule begins to develop. Eighth nerve has reached adult form. At $8\frac{1}{2}$ weeks, $2\frac{1}{2}$ turns of cochlea have developed. Cells that secrete tectorial membrane appear The lamina stapedialis appears. Ninth week: tympanic ring forms. |

TABLE 2. *Continued.*

Week of development (fertilization age)	10	12	14
Facial nerve	In weeks 10–11, the facial nerve branches extensively and some divisions reach the midline. In eleventh week, external petrosal nerve is present and VII communicates with V, IX, and X. Auricular branch of vagus reaches external auditory canal. All but four anastomoses of VII are present. Temporal division reaches frontalis. Small branches reach eyelids. Nasal muscles differentiate. By 80 mm, complex connections between superficial and deep portions of parotid primordium are present. Despite extensive branching, the vertical portion is still more anterior with respect to the external ear than in the adult (Figs. 41–45).		

External ear		Hillocks fuse to form auricle (Fig. 49).	
Middle ear	Pneumatization begins. Stapes changes ring shape to stirrup shape.	Twelfth to 28th week has four primary mucosal sacs emerge: saccus anticus—anterior pouch of von Tröltsch; saccus medius—epitympanum and petrous area; saccus superior—posterior pouch of von Tröltsch, part of mastoid, inferior incudal space; saccus posterior—round window and oval window niches, sinus tympani.	
Inner ear	Macular cell types are apparent and otolithic membrane is being formed. Capulae appear. Otoconia appear. Eleventh week, vestibular end-organs are formed. Tectorial membrane appears.	Scala tympani develops its space. Perichondrium of otic capsule appears. Eleventh to 12th week, fissula ante fenestram and fossula post fenestram develop.	Fourteen to 16 weeks, macular structures are well formed and similar to adults.

TABLE 2. *Continued.*

Week of development (fertilization age)	15	16	18
Facial nerve	Geniculate ganglion fully developed. Vertical portion of facial nerve still superficial with respect to future ear canal and mastoid cortex (Fig. 47).	All definitive communications of VII established. From weeks 16–20, VII and stapedius lie in sulcus that is differentiating from mesenchyme to connective tissue. VII moving toward adult position, but still anterior in middle ear and superficial with respect to ear canal (Fig. 50).	
External ear	Tympanic ring almost fully developed.	Auricular components recognizable but bulky (Fig. 61).	
Middle ear		Ossicles reach adult size. Ossification appears first at the long process of the incus. On 17th week, ossification centers become visible on the medial surface of the neck of the malleus, spreading to the manubrium and head.	Stapes ossification begins at the obturator surface of the stapedial base.
Inner ear	Formation of the membranous labyrinth is complete without the end-organ. First of the 14 centers of ossification can be identified. Scala vestibuli develops its space.		

Week of development (fertilization age)	20	21	22
Facial nerve	Facial nerve course is still more anterior and superficial than in the adult (Fig. 52).		
External ear	Auricle reaches adult shape (reaches adult size at about 9 years) (Fig. 62).	Epithelial core begins to resorb to form ear canal. Innermost layer remains as superficial layer of tectorial membrane.	
Middle ear			Antrum appears.
Inner ear	Stria vascularis and tectorial membrane are completed. Last of the 14 centers of ossification appears.		Fissula ante fenestram begins ossification.

TABLE 2. *Continued.*

Week of development (fertilization age)	23	26	28
Facial nerve		Sulcus partially closes and ossifies to become fallopian canal. Deep surface is completed first.	
External ear		Sixth month: Darwinian tubercle may appear.	Ear canal open (resorption complete).
Middle ear			Eardrum appears, derived from: ectoderm—squamous layer mesoderm—fibrous layer entoderm—mucosal layer. Stapes ossification is complete except vestibular surface of footplate.
Inner ear	Ossification of otic capsule is completed. Last area to ossify is the fissula ante fenestram (may remain cartilaginous throughout life). Membranous and bony labyrinth are adult size except for endolymphatic sac, which grows until adulthood. The two ridges divide: inner ridge cells become spiral limbus; outer ridge cells become hair cells, pillar cells, Hensen's cells, Deiters' cells. Bony spiral lamina develops.	Tunnel of Corti and space of Nuel are formed. Sixth month: inner spiral sulcus, inner and outer tunnels, and basilar membrane develop.	

Week of development (fertilization age)	30	35	Birth
Facial nerve	Normal relationship between ear canal, middle ear, and facial nerve established. Exit of the nerve through the stylomastoid foramen remains superficial until mastoid tip develops between ages one and three years.	Geniculate ganglion separated from epitympanum by bone.	In about two-thirds, some or all mandibular branches are below the angle of the mandible. Mandibular branches are above mandibular margin as they cross the facial artery. Fallopian canal fully developed, but dehiscent in about 25%.
External ear	Excavation of the tympanic cavity is complete.		Shape of auricle complete, but continues to grow until age nine. Ear canal not ossified. Ossification complete at about age three. Size reached at about age nine.
Middle ear			Middle ear is well formed. It enlarges only slightly after birth. Middle ear is partially still filled with mucoid connective tissue. It is resorbed within a few months and pneumatization of middle ear, antrum, and mastoid continues. Pneumatization of petrous portion arises last and continues until puberty.

TABLE 2. *Continued.*

Week of development (fertilization age)	30	35	Birth
			Mastoid process appears at age one, not formed until about age three.
			Tympanic ring and ear canal are ossified at age three.
			Eustachian tube is 17 mm at birth and grows to 36 mm.
			Malleus, incus, and stapes are adult size and shape.
			Part of manubrium of malleus remains cartilaginous and never ossifies. Vestibular surface of stapes never ossifies. Petrous, squamous, and tympanic ring portions of temporal bone are distinguishable, and styloid process is recognizable.
Inner ear			Membranous and bony labyrinth are adult size except endolymphatic sac, which grows until adulthood (first structure to appear and last to stop growing).

The only other systematic, chronological correlation of ear and facial nerve embryology was published in 1986 by Schuknecht and Gulya (56). Although it is excellent and presents a chronological discussion of ear embryology similar to that constructed for this study, it provides only a limited summary of facial nerve development, as appropriate in the context in which it appears. A more complete description of comparative embryology of the ear and facial nerve has not been published heretofore. The descriptions of embryology of the ear presented in the following discussion are common knowledge and have been described previously in numerous sources and standard texts (56, 61– 65). Because of the publication of the book by Schuknecht and Gulya (56) which presents embryology of the ear in such a convenient fashion, the discussion of that subject in this book has been condensed to briefly summarize information about facial nerve development essential for clinical application. Following the description of comparative embryology of the ear and facial nerve, the findings are reduced to a summary table. This has proven convenient in allowing the surgeon to review readily the expected status and position of *all* otologic and facial nerve structures if any *one* of them can be observed.

To test the validity of this approach, observations were made during surgery on 13 malformed ears of eleven patients cared for by the author. The thorough description of facial nerve embryology presented and its correlation with known information about embryology of the ear have been helpful and appear to be valuable in preparing the otologist for surgery on malformed ears.

The literature on embryology of the facial nerve describes specimens in terms of crown-rump length, fetal age, or menstrual age. For the purposes of this discussion, all reports have been converted to fertilization age using standard conversion tables (66–68) (Tables 1 and 2).

ADULT ANATOMY

In studying embryology of the facial nerve, it is helpful to keep in mind the final structure toward which development is directed. In the adult, the motor nucleus of the facial nerve is deep in the reticu-

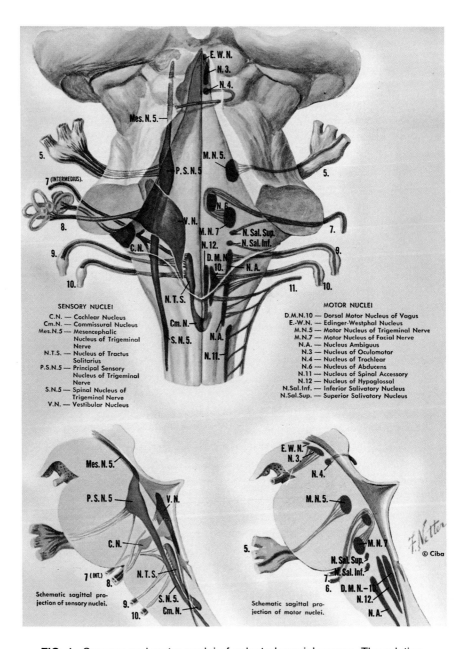

FIG. 1. Sensory and motor nuclei of selected cranial nerves. The relationship of the seventh nerve and its nuclei to surrounding structures is illustrated. (From ref. 71) © Copyright 1983 CIBA-GEIGY Corporation. Reprinted with permission from THE CIBA COLLECTION OF MEDICAL ILLUSTRATIONS, illustrated by Frank H. Netter, M.D. All rights reserved.

lar formation of the caudal portion of the pons (Fig. 1). The axons leave the motor nucleus extending dorsally and medially (cranially and superficially), and they bend around the abducens nucleus, forming the first genu of the facial nerve. The fibers then course deep through the pons to exit from the central nervous system between the olive and inferior cerebellar peduncle. At this point, the axons join to form the motor root. The sensory root is called the nervus intermedius and consists of central processes of neurons located in the geniculate ganglion and axons of parasympathetic neurons from the superior salivatory nucleus. The nervus intermedius enters the central nervous system at the pontocerebellar groove lateral to the motor root, and synapses with neurons in the upper part of the tractus solitarius. The facial nerve and nervus intermedius course with the vestibuloacoustic nerve from the brain stem to enter the internal auditory canal (Fig. 2). Approximately 20% of the time the nervus intermedius is fused with the eighth cranial nerve (46).

Once the facial nerve enters the middle ear, it bends a second time at the geniculate ganglion (the second genu) and courses horizontally through the middle ear (Fig. 3). It then curves (the pyramidal bend) to course vertically through the mastoid bone and exit at the stylomastoid foramen (Fig. 4). The nerve is ordinarily surrounded by a bony sheath called the fallopian canal. Several branches are given off during the intrapetrosal course. The facial nerve spreads extratemporally to supply the facial musculature (Fig. 5).

From medial to lateral, the facial nerve branches include (Fig. 6): (a) Communications in the internal auditory canal with the eighth cranial nerve. (b) The greater superficial petrosal nerve, which supplies taste fibers to the anterior two-thirds of the tongue, preganglionic parasympathetic fibers to the submandibular gland, and the lacrimal gland, nasal glands, and palatine mucosal glands. It also communicates with the lesser petrosal nerve (46). (c) The nerve to the stapedius muscle. (d) The chorda tympani nerve, which supplies taste fibers to the anterior two-thirds of the tongue, preganglionic parasympathetic fibers to the submandibular gland, and postganglionic fibers to the submandibular and sublingual glands. (e) The posterior auricular branch, which innervates the auricularis posterior, cranially-oriented muscles of the auricle, and the occipital

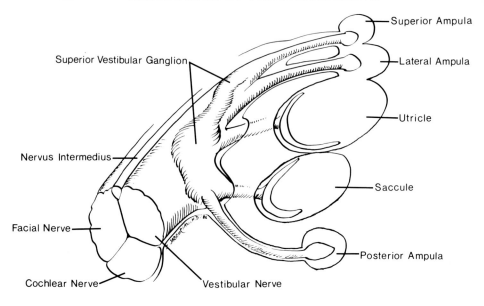

FIG. 2. The usual relationships of the seventh and eighth cranial nerves as they enter the internal auditory canal and temporal bone.

muscles. It communicates with the greater auricular nerve, auricular branch of the vagus nerve, and lesser occipital nerve (50). (f) The branch to the posterior belly of the digastric muscle. (g) The branch to the stylohyoid muscle. (h) The temporal branch, which supplies the lateral intrinsic muscle of the auricle, the anterior, and superior auricular muscles, and the frontalis, orbicularis oculi, and corruga-tor muscles. (i) The buccal branch, which innervates the procerus, zygomaticus major, levator labii superioris alaeque nasi, levator an-guli oris, zygomaticus minor, nasal muscles, buccinator, and or-bicularis oris. (j) The marginal mandibular branch to the risorius and muscles of the lower lip and chin. (k) The cervical branch to the platysma. There are interconnections between the facial nerve and primary sensory nerves including the trigeminal, glossopharyngeal, vagus, and cervical nerves (50).

The intracranial portion of the facial nerve is supplied by the ante-rior inferior cerebellar artery (Figs. 7 and 8). The intrapetrosal por-tion is supplied by the superficial petrosal branch of the middle

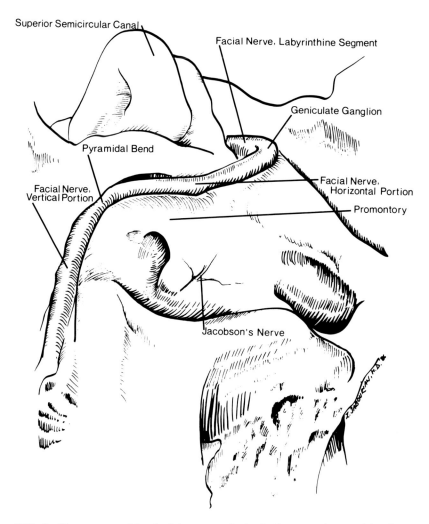

FIG. 3. The course of the facial nerve anterior to the superior semicircular canal, and in its horizontal course through the middle ear.

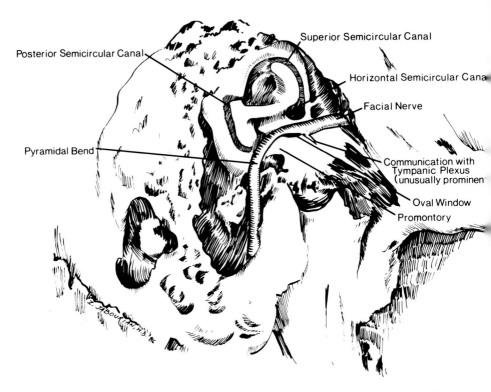

FIG. 4. The relationship of the facial nerve in its horizontal and vertical portions to other temporal bone landmarks.

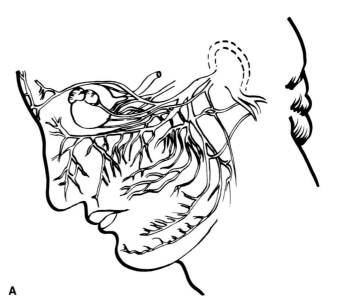

A

FIG. 5. A: The distribution of the facial nerve to muscles of the face after the nerve has exited from the stylomastoid foramen. The extratemporal anatomy of the facial nerve is variable. **FIG. 5.** *Continues.*

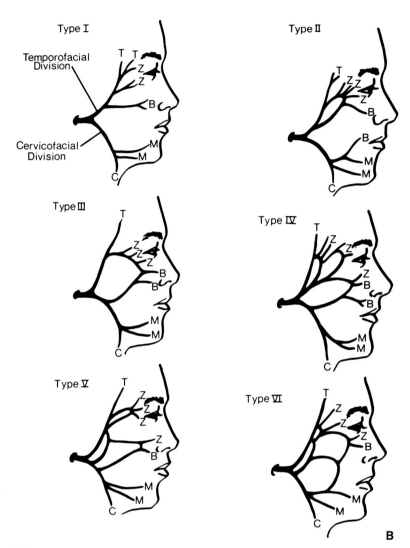

FIG. 5. *Continued.* **B:** Common patterns of branching of the extracranial portion of the facial nerve. Type I is seen in 20% of cases; type II, in 37.5%; type III, in 20%; type IV, in 15%; type V, in 15%; and type VI, in 2.5%, according to Coker and Fisch. T, Temporal branch; Z, Zygomatic branch; B, Buccal branch; M, Marginal mandibular branch; C, Cervical branch. (Modified from ref. 72, with permission.)

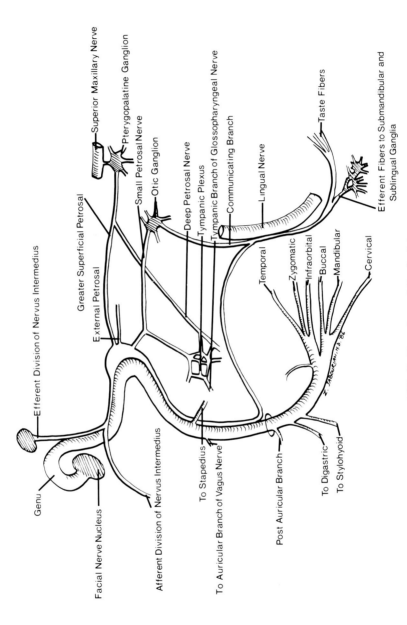

FIG. 6. Branches of the facial nerve.

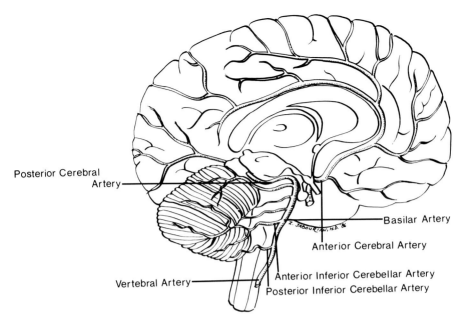

Posterior Cerebral Artery

Basilar Artery

Anterior Cerebral Artery

Anterior Inferior Cerebellar Artery

Vertebral Artery

Posterior Inferior Cerebellar Artery

FIG. 7. Origin of the anterior inferior cerebellar artery, which supplies blood to the intracranial portion of the facial nerve.

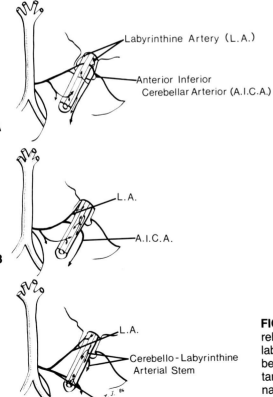

Labyrinthine Artery (L.A.)

Anterior Inferior Cerebellar Arterior (A.I.C.A.)

A

L.A.

A.I.C.A.

B

L.A.

Cerebello-Labyrinthine Arterial Stem

A.I.C.A.

FIG. 8. The anterior inferior cerebellar artery also gives off the labyrinthine artery. Its origin may be within **(A)**, close to **(B)**, or distant from the internal auditory canal **(C)**. (Modified from ref. 73, with permission.)

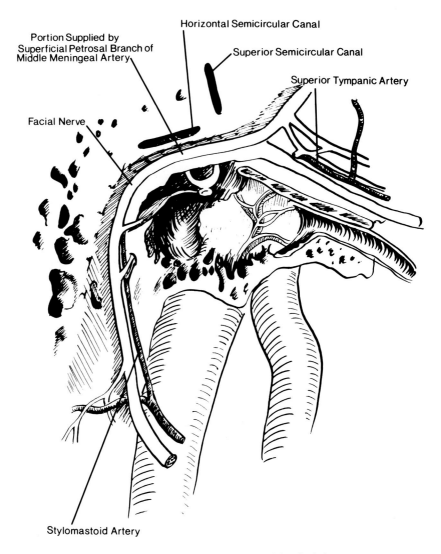

FIG. 9. Intratemporal blood supply of the facial nerve.

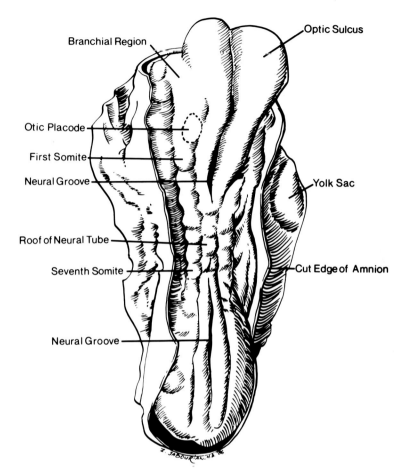

FIG. 10. The dorsum of a seven-somite human embryo (approximately 22 days old). (Modified from ref. 59, with permission.)

meningeal artery and the stylomastoid branch of the posterior auricular artery (Fig. 9). The extracranial portion is supplied by the stylomastoid, posterior auricular, superficial temporal, and transverse facial arteries. The anastomosis between the intratemporal branches usually occurs in the upper third of the vertical portion.

EMBRYOLOGY OF THE INTRACRANIAL PORTION
OF THE FACIAL NERVE

This book focuses primarily on the development of the extra-cranial portions of the facial nerve. Knowledge of this subject is useful in understanding congenital anomalies or diseases of the facial nerve and in planning surgery of the temporal bone and parotid gland. However, a brief review of the embryology of the intra-cranial portion of the facial nerve is helpful for orientation.

In the 22-day-old human embryo (seven somites), the otic placode can be seen in the narrow area between the bilobed region of the neural plate and the first somite (Fig. 10). This narrow region will form the mesencephalon and the rhombencephalon. By the ten-somite stage (about 23 days) the rhombencephalic region of the neural plate has closed into a tube. As the anterior neuropore is closed, the region of the brain shows three dilatations: the forebrain, the prosencephalic cavity; the midbrain, the mesencephalic cavity; and the hindbrain, rhombencephalic cavity. The constricted region joining the mesencephalon to the rhombencephalon is the isthmus, as can be seen in the 36-day embryo (9 mm) (Fig. 11). By approximately 40 days (11 mm), the rhombencephalon is subdivided into a caudal myelencephalon and a cranial metencephalon. The facial nerve exists between the metencephalon and the myelencephalon (Fig. 12). The deepening pontine flexure will become the fourth ventricle as can be seen easily in the nine-week embryo (Fig. 13).

The motor fibers of the facial nerve arrive near the floor of what will become the fourth ventricle, primarily from a nuclear group in the special visceral efferent column of the posterior portion of the metencephalon (Fig. 14). It used to be believed that sensory fibers associated with the geniculate ganglion arose from neuroblasts closely associated with the developing eighth cranial nerve in the acousticofacial primordium. It is now clear that the eighth cranial nerve develops from the anteromedial aspect of the otic placode, whereas the special visceral afferent fibers of the facial nerve (taste) arise independently from the acousticofacial primordium (26, 63). In the brain stem, the sixth and seventh cranial nerves develop in close proximity, as can be seen in the 45-day embryo (Fig. 15). A

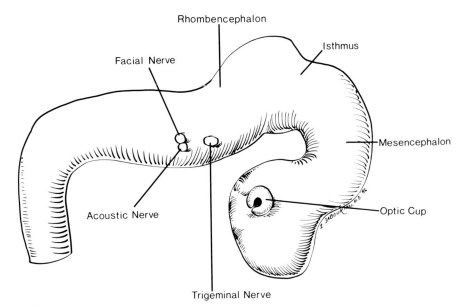

FIG. 11. External appearance of the right side of the central nervous system in a 36-day-old embryo (9 mm). The acoustic and facial nerves are distinct. (Modified from ref. 59, with permission.)

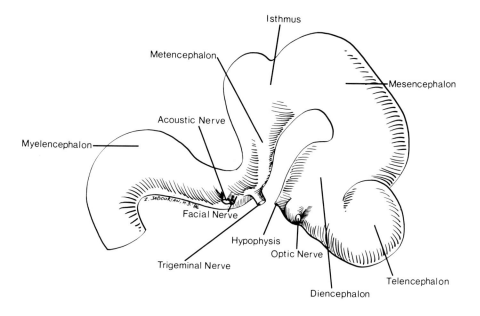

FIG. 12. A 40-day-old embryo illustrating the developing relationship between the facial nerve and acoustic nerve as the pontine flexure deepens. (Modified from ref. 59, with permission.)

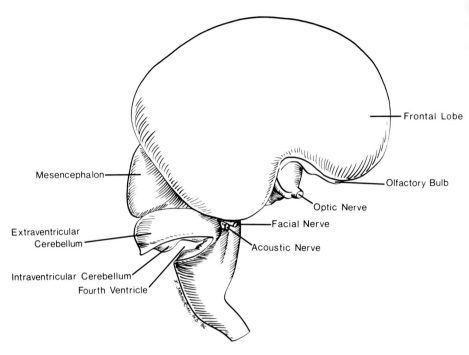

FIG. 13. The right half of the cranial portion of the central nervous system of a nine-week-old embryo (53 mm). The development of the pontine flexure into the fourth ventricle can be seen. (The roof of the fourth ventricle has been removed.) (Modified from ref. 59, with permission.)

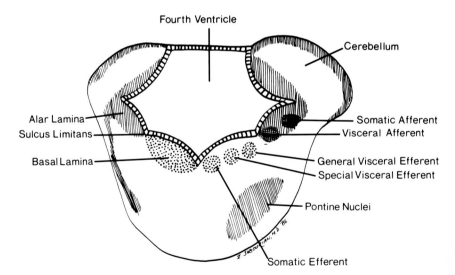

FIG. 14. The alar and basal laminae in the myelencephalon (medulla) and metencephalon (pons), and their development. The left half of the figure (on which the sulcus limitans is labeled) is at an earlier stage of development than the right half of the figure. (Modified from ref. 59, with permission.)

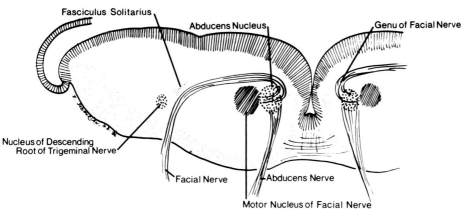

FIG. 15. A 6¹/₂-week-old embryo showing the development of the motor nuclei and roots of the sixth and seventh cranial nerves. The first genu of the facial nerve can also be identified as it bends around the nucleus of the sixth cranial nerve.

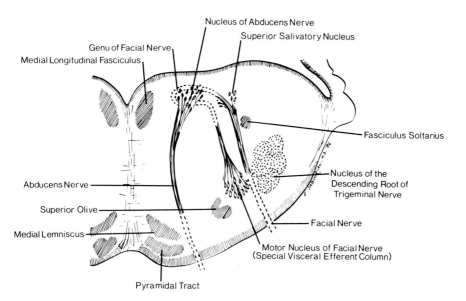

FIG. 16. In the eleven-week-old fetus, the relationships among the sixth and seventh cranial nerves and their nuclei in the brain stem resemble those of the adult.

more mature relationship is clear by eleven weeks (Fig. 16). As development proceeds, the myelencephalon will become the medulla oblongata, the site of attachment of cranial nerves IX through XII. The dorsal portion of the metencephalon will develop into the cerebellum.

PHYLOGENY

The phylogenetic origins of the ear have been beautifully summarized by Schuknecht and Gulya (56). The information they presented will not be restated here, so the reader is encouraged to consult their book. However, Schuknecht and Gulya did not discuss the phylogenetic origins of the facial nerve and muscles.

The phylogeny of the muscles of facial expression is somewhat less obvious than that of other muscles of branchiomeric origin. Most muscles retain the innervation appropriate to their gill-arch stages in phylogeny. For example, muscles that arise from the mandibular arch (temporalis, masseter, pterygoids, anterior belly of the digastric, tensor veli palantini, mylohyoid, and tensor tympani) are supplied by the trigeminal nerve, the nerve of the mandibular arch. This seems logical. However, this arrangement preempts the muscles of the mandibular arch region for use in chewing and swallowing. In lower life forms up through fish, facial expression is limited to mandibular motion. Since there is no muscle tissue between the skin and bones in the face of the fish and muscles of chewing and swallowing are not available for facial expression, the hyoid arch provides the nearest available muscle. Consequently, muscles of the hyoid region migrate to permit facial expression. As animals increase in complexity from fish to amphibia to mammals, the extent of hyoid arch muscle migration into the face also increases. In amphibia an outer superficial layer of muscle in the former gill area acts as a primitive constrictor. In mammals, both deep and superficial layers of hyoid musculature spread into the face carrying the facial nerve with them and creating its intricate course (Fig. 17). We see this process recapitulated in the developing human embryo in the sixth and seventh weeks (58). The frontalis, auricularis, occipitalis, and platysma colli muscles are derived from the primordial

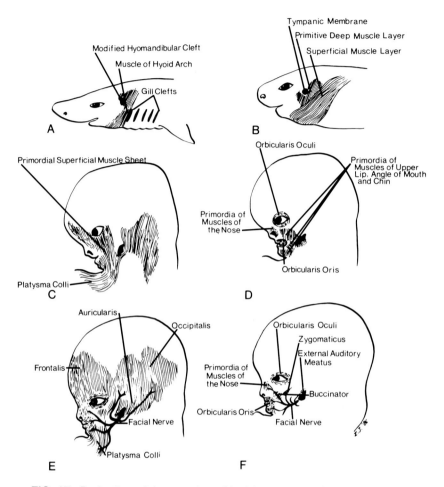

FIG. 17. Derivation of the muscles of facial expression from migration and differentiation of hyoid arch musculature. **A:** Location of hyoid arch muscles in fish. **B:** An additional sheet of superficial muscle appears in some amphibia. **C:** A primordial superficial muscle sheet appears in human embryos at six weeks. **D:** The primordial deep muscle layer becomes organized into musculature around the mouth and nose during the sixth week. **E:** Superficial muscles of the head are developed by the seventh week. **F:** Deep muscles of the face appear at seven weeks. (Modified from ref. 58, with permission.)

superficial muscle sheet. The primordial deep layer of muscle from the hyoid arch gives rise to muscles controlling movements of the nose, lips, and around the eye. Recognizing the migration of these muscles and the facial nerve, as well as branches of the external carotid artery they carry with them is helpful in understanding the complex anatomy of the human adult and the congenitally abnormal anatomy associated with interrupted migration during development.

FERTILIZATION THROUGH THE FOURTH WEEK

The Facial Nerve

The facioacoustic primordium appears during the third week of life. It is attached to the metencephalon just rostral to the otic vesicle. It is fibrous at its attachment but becomes more cellular ventrally, more compact, and appears as a column of cells (44). It becomes more superficial and rostral as it proceeds ventrally, and it ends adjacent to the deep surface of the epibranchial placode on the dorsal and caudal aspect of the first branchial groove. There are no branches, and the geniculate ganglion is not yet present (Fig. 18). Later in the fourth week, by the time the embryo reaches 4.8 mm, the facial nerve splits into two parts. The chorda tympani nerve comes off rostrally and courses ventrally to the first pharyngeal pouch to enter the mandibular arch. The caudal main trunk disappears in mesenchyme (Fig. 19). By the time the embryo is 6 mm in length, the nerve approaches the epibranchial placode and large, dark nuclei mark the development of the geniculate ganglion (44).

The Ear

The primordium of the membranous labyrinth is the first part of the ear to appear. This makes sense, as it is phylogenetically the oldest ear structure, and it heralds the development of the balance system that is so essential for survival of lower life forms. Early in the third week (two-somite stage) a thickening appears in the super-

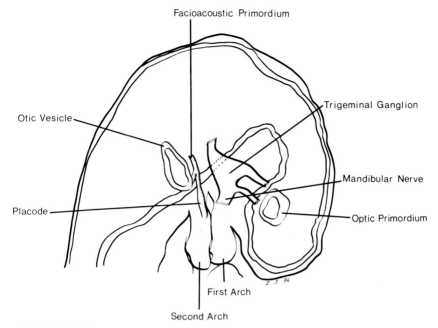

FIG. 18. A 4.2-mm embryo approximately 3½ weeks old. The region of the epibranchial placode of the second arch is labeled. (Modified from ref. 44, with permission.)

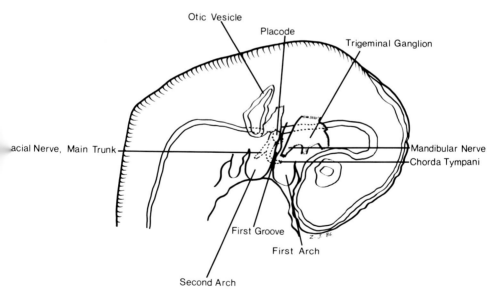

FIG. 19. A 4.8-mm embryo approximately 4½ weeks old. At this stage, neuroblasts of the developing geniculate and acoustic ganglia have developed. This embryo is somewhat more developed than expected for its length. (Modified from ref. 44, with permission.)

ficial ectoderm on both sides of the neural plate. This thickening is the otic placode. It becomes clearly marked by the middle of the third week. The otic placode develops in conjunction with the acousticofacial ganglion lateral to the rhombencephalon. The acousticofacial ganglion cells extend downward ventrally as far as the second epibranchial placode. Taste fibers of the facial nerve arise from the second branchial arch. The eighth nerve arises from cells of the auditory placode.

While the inner ear is making its initial appearance, the first and second pouches may be found lateral to the primordium of the oral and pharyngeal tongue. As the third arch enlarges, the space between the second arch and the pharynx is compressed, becoming the eustachian tube. An out-pocketing of the lateral end of the first pouch becomes the middle ear space. Throughout the fourth and fifth week, the pouch moves more laterally toward the first branchial groove. It later constricts to become recognizable as the eustachian tube and middle ear space.

During the fourth week, the otic placode invaginates to become the otic pit. Then the surface opening closes, making it the otocyst or otic vesicle. Otic placode cells migrate to the otic vesicle basement membrane to reach the area where the auditory nerve ganglion will form. During this period, the common macula also appears, and angiogenesis around the otic vesicle begins. As the first pouch continues to migrate laterally, a condensation of mesenchyme appears during the fourth week. This condensation is the stapes blastema. The facial nerve divides the blastema into the stapes, interhyale, and laterohyale. The structures formed by the laterohyale and interhyale will be seen at about eight weeks. The facial nerve establishes relationships important later in development (Fig. 20). Initially, it divides the stapes blastema into the laterohyale and stapes, connected by the interhyale. During development, the structures appear to rotate about the facial nerve so that the laterohyale eventually will lie posterior to the stapes. This is owing to the inferior expansion of the laterohyale primordium and the superior expansion of the stapes. The blastemae of the malleus and incus lie on both sides of the first branchial groove. This observation helps explain their branchial arch origin, which appears confusing when only the adult structures are observed. The chorda tympani nerve bends

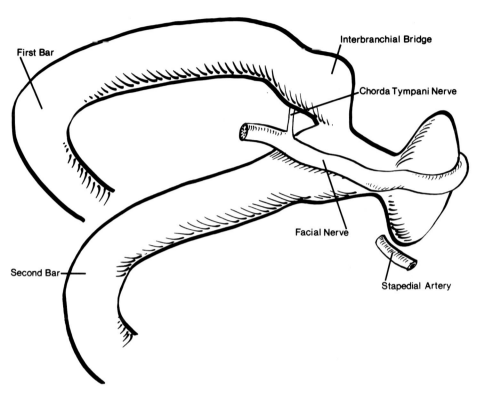

FIG. 20. Configuration of the visceral bars at 4½ weeks (7 mm) illustrating the relationship of the facial nerve to the precursors of ear structures. (Modified from ref. 63, with permission.)

around the ventral aspect of the interbranchial bridge (incus and malleus primordia). As a slower-growing structure, it will provide a fixed point about which the malleus and incus will develop.

FIFTH THROUGH SIXTH WEEK

The Facial Nerve

By the time the embryo has reached 7 mm in length near the beginning of the fifth week, the mesenchymal concentrations that form the cephalic muscles can be seen in association with their nerves (Fig. 21). The geniculate ganglion and nervus intermedius also appear, although the nervus intermedius may not be visible as a separate nerve until approximately the seventh week (44). The geniculate ganglion is lateral and rostral to the eighth nerve ganglion. The greater superficial petrosal nerve is present. The chorda tympani is large and enters the mandibular arch, terminating near a branch of the mandibular nerve that will become the lingual nerve. By the middle of the fifth week (10 mm), the facial nerve gives off small branches to the posterior digastric premuscle mass. The nerve terminates in mesenchyme.

In the 8-mm embryo, all of the cranial nerves except the olfactory nerve and optic nerve are recognizable. All of the cranial nerves carrying sensory fibers have prominent ganglia near their points of connection with the brain. These include cranial nerves V, VII, VIII, IX, and X. Primarily efferent cranial nerves (III, IV, VI, and XII) have no external ganglia (Fig. 22).

In the 8- to 14-mm period, the posterior auricular nerve appears near the chorda tympani. Complete separation of the facial and acoustic nerves is apparent, and a discrete nervus intermedius develops. By 14 mm, the geniculate ganglion and the greater superficial petrosal nerve are well defined, and the epibranchial placode has disappeared (Fig. 23). The greater superficial petrosal nerve courses ventrally and rostrally to the lateral aspect of the developing internal carotid artery. Here it joins the deep petrosal nerve and continues as the nerve of the pterygoid canal. It terminates in a group of cells that will become the pterygopalatine ganglion. At 16 to 17 mm (late in the sixth week), a branch arises from the ventral aspect of the geniculate ganglion and courses caudally and dorsally to the glossopharyngeal ganglion. The chorda tympani and lingual nerves end near the developing submandibular ganglion. Some facial nerve fibers terminate in the mandibular arch superficially and caudally. During this period (Fig. 24), the superficial layer of the second arch mesenchymal lamina spreads to establish (a) occipital lamina (occipitalis, auricularis posterior, transversus nuchae muscles), (b) cervical lamina (cervical part of platysma), (c) mandibular lamina (depressor labii inferioris, mentalis, risorius, depressor anguli oris, inferior part of the orbicularis oris, and possibly the buccinator and levator anguli oris), and (d) temporal lamina (auricularis superior), which spreads in the latter part of this stage. The deep

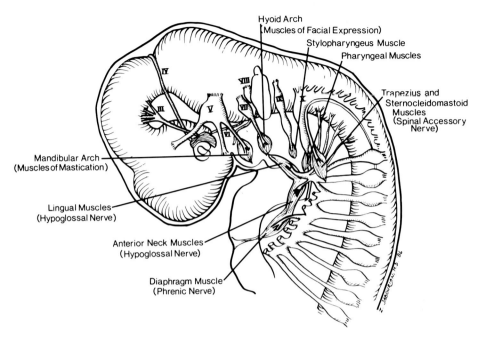

FIG. 21. Diagram of a 4½-week-old embryo illustrating the mesenchymal concentrations that will give rise to the cephalic muscles, as well as the cranial nerves associated with them. (Modified from ref. 58, with permission.)

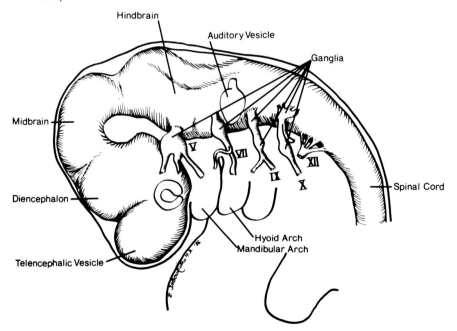

FIG. 22. Development of the cranial nerves and ganglia in an embryo slightly over five weeks old (8 mm). (Modified from ref. 58, with permission.)

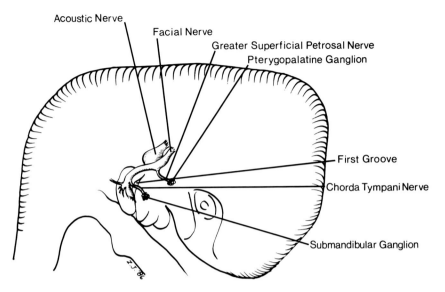

FIG. 23. Further development of the facial nerve and its relationship to the acoustic nerve is seen in this six-week-old embryo (14 mm). (Modified from ref. 44, with permission.)

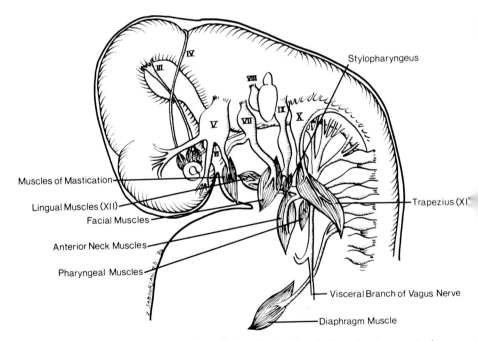

FIG. 24. A six-week-old embryo (11 mm) showing further development of the premuscle masses of the cephalic muscles. (Modified from ref. 58, with permission.)

layer of the second mesenchymal lamina differentiates into the posterior digastric complex (stapedius, posterior belly of the digastric,
digastric tendon, and stylohyoid muscles) (10–18 mm).

The Ear

At the end of the fourth week and the beginning of the fifth week,
the pharyngeal pouch entoderm and the ectoderm of the floor of the

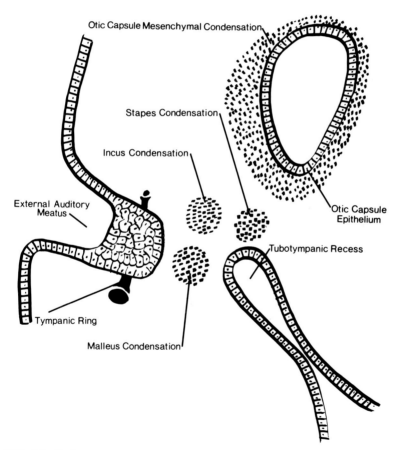

FIG. 25. Embryo approximately five weeks in age showing the development of the tubotympanic recess and primordial masses of the ossicles.

first branchial groove (gill furrow) are in contact for a short period of time. The blind end of the first pouch constitutes the primordium of the tympanic cavity, and it pulls away from the surface. The concentration of mesenchyme adjacent to it is the primordial mass of the ossicles (Fig. 25). The first branchial groove (first gill furrow) constitutes the primordium of the external auditory meatus. The ossicles develop above the primordial tympanic cavity. Apparent rotation of the developing ear structures around the facial nerves continues (Fig. 26).

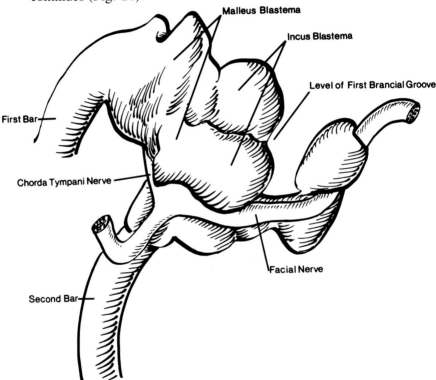

FIG. 26. A 5½-week-old embryo showing further apparent rotation of the primordial middle ear structures around the facial nerve. (Modified from ref. 63, with permission.)

In the fifth week, as the auditory vesicle enlarges, it changes from its original spheroidal shape to become elongated. It develops a wide dorsal and slender ventral portion. Between them, the endolymphatic duct and sac emerge at about the point at which the otic vesicle separated from the superficial ectoderm. The dorsal portion will become the vestibular part of the labyrinth; the ventral portion, the cochlear part of the labyrinth. Concurrently, at the end of the fourth and the beginning of the fifth weeks, the acoustic ganglion divides into a superior (vestibular) and inferior (cochlear) structure. Simultaneously, a mesenchymal condensation marks the beginning of the otic capsule.

During the sixth week, the semicircular canals appear. At this time, the common macula is differentiated. Its superior (upper) part forms the utricular macula and the cristae of the superior and lateral semicircular canals. The inferior (lower) part forms the saccular macula and the crista of the posterior semicircular canal. The mesenchyme forming the otic capsule takes on a cartilaginous appearance. This cartilage is the anlage of enchondral bone, the hardest bone in the body. Along with a thin layer of endosteal bone, it will surround completely the membranous labyrinth. Following formation of the semicircular canals during the sixth week, tissue is absorbed leading to the characteristic appearance of the canals.

The auricle develops as tissue growth of the first and second branchial arches around the dorsal extremity of the first branchial groove. Differentiation in this area is first noticeable at around four weeks. However, the precursors of the auricle are not prominent until the sixth week. At this time, mesoderm of the first and second arches condenses to form the six hillocks of His (Fig. 27). Controversies remain unresolved regarding the importance of these hillocks and their homologues (56). The scheme described by Pearson and Jacobson (63) appears reasonable. They suggest that the first arch develops into the first three hillocks. The first hillock forms the tragus. The second hillock forms the helical crus. The third hillock forms the helix. The second arch provides the fourth, fifth, and sixth hillocks. The fourth hillock forms the antihelix. The fifth forms the antitragus. The sixth forms the lobule and lower helix. The conchae forms from three areas of first-groove ectoderm. The middle part of the first groove forms the concha cavum. The upper

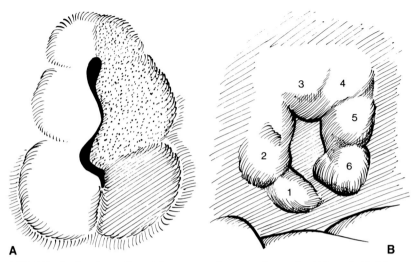

FIG. 27. A: Configuration of the external ear at six weeks (13 mm). **B:** The six hillocks of His are believed to fuse to form the developing auricle.

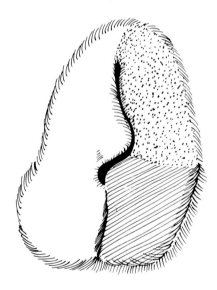

FIG. 28. At 6½ weeks (17 mm) the hillocks are less distinct and further apart.

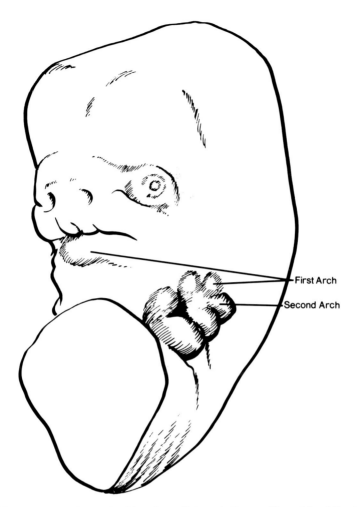

FIG. 29. In the six-week-old embryo (14 mm), the position of the hillocks of His can be seen in relationship to the other developing structures of the head.

part forms the concha cymba. The lower part forms the intertragus incisura.

During the sixth week, the hillocks are pushed further apart by development of the first groove (Fig. 28). By the end of the sixth week, the hillocks have given rise to the two folds of the developing auricle. Fusion of the two folds takes place at the upper end of the branchial groove. The developing ears are positioned low and laterally (Figs. 29 and 30). In the adult, the regions derived from hill-

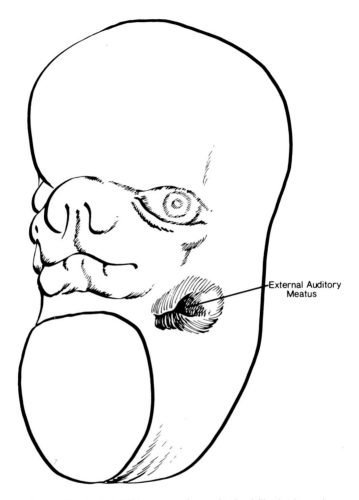

External Auditory
Meatus

FIG. 30. By the beginning of the seventh week, the hillocks have begun to fuse, and the developing external auditory meatus has begun to rotate toward its adult position. However, at this stage, it is still low with respect to its final position.

ocks one, two, and three are innervated by the auriculotemporal branch of the trigeminal nerve (nerve of the mandibular arch). The structures derived from hillocks four, five, and six are innervated by the greater auricular nerve, lesser occipital nerve, and cutaneous sensory branches of the facial nerve (nerve of the hyoid arch).

SEVENTH THROUGH NINTH WEEK

The Facial Nerve

By the beginning of the seventh week, the embryo has reached approximately 18 mm in length (Fig. 31). The nervus intermedius is smaller than the motor root of the facial nerve and passes into the brain stem between the acoustic nerve and the facial nerve motor root. The chorda tympani and lingual nerves unite proximal to the submandibular gland. The postauricular nerve can be seen clearly, distal to the chorda tympani nerves, and divides into cranial and caudal branches. The caudal branches communicate with branches of C-2 and C-3. Several branches are visible in the peripheral portion of the seventh nerve. The most caudal branches communicate with nerves from the second and third cervical ganglia in a plexus in the second arch. Another portion courses ventrally, terminating deep to the platysma myoblastic lamina. The rest of the branches course to the angle of the mouth or caudally and superiorly into the mandibular arch. By 19 mm, some branches have reached the infra-

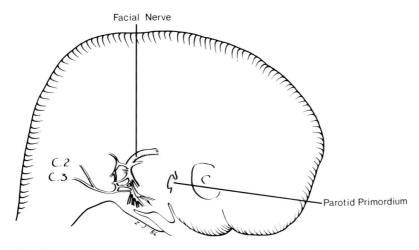

FIG. 31. An 18-mm embryo approximately seven weeks of age. The horizontal and vertical portions of the facial nerve can be identified, and facial nerve branching has developed. Anastomoses with C-2 and C-3 are also seen. (Modified from ref. 44, with permission.)

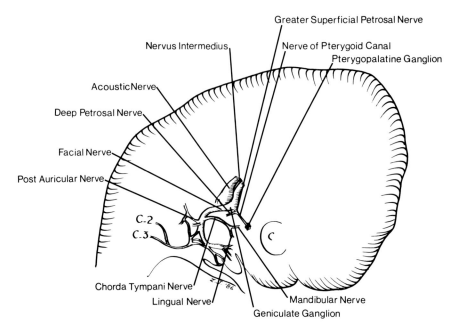

FIG. 32. The relationship between the facial nerve and parotid primordium at approximately seven weeks (18 mm). (Modified from ref. 48, with permission.)

orbital rim. All of the peripheral branches lie close to the deep surfaces of the myoblastic laminae that will form facial muscles. Very few fibers course dorsally. The zygomatic and temporal nerves will arise from higher in the facial nerve. At 18 mm, the parotid bud is rostral and unbranched, appearing as an evagination from the lateral oral cavity area (Fig. 32).

In the 22-mm embryo (middle of the seventh week), the posterior belly of the digastric, the stapedius, and the stylohyoid muscles are developing (Fig. 33). A branch from the geniculate ganglion near the greater superficial petrosal nerve that developed earlier is reduced to a communication as the tympanic plexus and lesser petrosal nerve develop from the ninth cranial nerve. The interanastamoses of the peripheral branches of the facial nerve are visible as separations of the main trunk. A small nerve branch approaches the buccal region superficial to the parotid bud (Fig. 34).

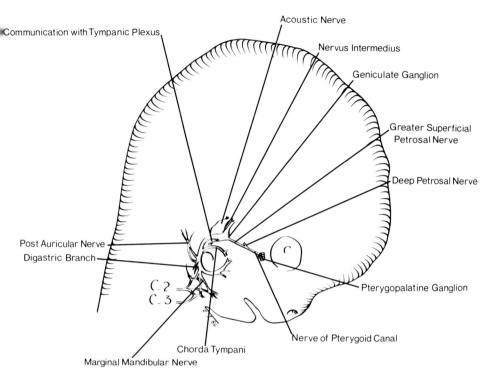

FIG. 33. By the middle of the seventh week (22 mm), additional branching has occurred. However, the structures of the facial nerve are still anterior with respect to the external auditory meatus, which is in the process of migration from its original location low on the developing embryo (see Fig. 30). (Modified from ref. 44, with permission.)

Separations between nerve branches increase considerably in number and size by the end of the seventh week (26 mm) (Fig. 35). The branch to the stapedius muscle is visible. This branch is probably present in earlier specimens but can only be visualized after the branch separates from the main trunk when the embryo reaches 26 mm in length (44). Peripheral branches course cranially to become the zygomatic and temporal divisions. The buccal, mandibular, and cervical divisions constitute approximately one-half of the peripheral branches. All of the peripheral divisions can be identified, but the temporal branches have not yet reached the frontal region.

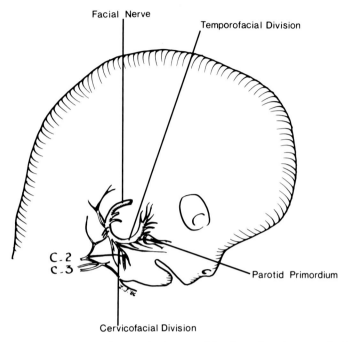

FIG. 34. At 7¹/₂ weeks (22 mm), the parotid primordium has reached the distal branches of the developing facial nerve. The temporofacial and cervicofacial divisions can be identified. (Modified from ref. 48, with permission.)

Anastomoses are well established with the infraorbital, buccal, auriculotemporal, and mental branches of the trigeminal nerve. Previously established communications with branches of C-2 and C-3 have become communications with the greater auricular and transverse cervical nerves. A combined marginal mandibular-cervical branch is present between 20 and 45 mm (seventh through middle of the eighth week), the superficial layer of the second arch mesenchyme differentiates into two more laminae (50): (a) infraorbital (zygomaticus major and minor, levator labii superioris alaeque nasi, the superior part of the orbicularis oris, possibly the compressor naris, depressor septi, orbicularis oculi, frontalis, corrugator supercilii, and procerus); and (b) occipital platysma.

Between 24 and 26 mm, the zygomaticus major, depressor anguli oris, and buccinator appear. Between 27 and 45 mm, the frontalis

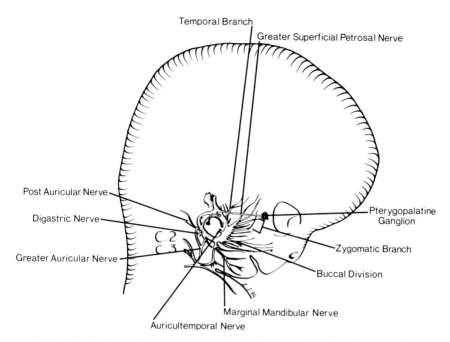

FIG. 35. As the embryo approaches the eighth week (26 mm), separations can be seen between nerve branches. The branches have also increased in size and number. (Modified from ref. 44, with permission.)

and zygomaticus minor appear. The branch connecting VII with the lesser petrosal nerve (from cranial nerve IX) apparently carries small myelinated fibers with interspersed autonomic fibers from the auricular branch of X. In addition, by 26 mm the embryo also reveals development of first-order ductules of the parotid primordium. It lies next to the masseter muscle, and several branches of the facial nerve course superficial to it (48). By 27 mm, second-order ductules appear. At this time, the buccal, marginal mandibular, and cervical nerve branches approach the parotid primordium. By 32 mm (eighth week), third-order ductules are present and the primordium has entered the parotid space. In the 37-mm fetus (8½ weeks), fourth-order parotid ductules are present, and buccal nerve branches are superficial to the main duct (Fig. 36). The temporal, zygomatic, and upper buccal branches are superficial on the parotid primordium. The lower buccal, mandibular, and cervical branches are deeper.

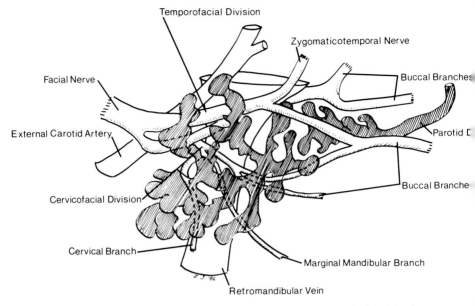

FIG. 36. During the eighth week (37-mm fetus) complex relationships between the facial nerve and parotid primordium are established. The temporofacial branches are more superficial than the cervicofacial branches, and the buccal branches are superficial to the parotid duct. (Modified from ref. 48, with permission.)

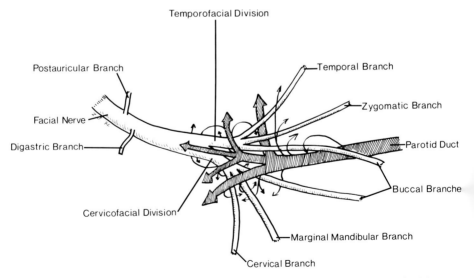

FIG. 37. The pattern of development of the parotid gland around the facial nerve and its branches. (Modified from ref. 48, with permission.)

The postauricular nerve goes to the occipital region and a branch to the dorsal aspect of the auricle is present. Although there are no branches to the fused eyelids yet, a branch from the temporal division approaches the frontal region. The progressive directional relationship between the parotid gland and facial nerve was illustrated most clearly by Gasser (48) (Fig. 37).

During the eighth week, a sulcus develops around the facial nerve, blood vessels, and stapedius muscle on the posterior aspect of the cartilaginous otic capsule. The sulcus is the beginning of the fallopian canal. The orbicularis oris, levator anguli oris, and orbicularis oculi muscles also appear at around 37 mm (50). During the ninth week (50 to 60 mm), the auricularis anterior, corrugator supercilii, occipital and mandibular platysma, and levator labii superioris muscles appear. About the ninth week, the laterohyale fuses to the otic capsule to form part of the anterior wall of the fallopian canal and the pyramidal eminence. The segment of the anterior wall of the fallopian canal distal to the laterohyale is formed by Reichert's cartilage. The cranial nerves move closer to their adult relationships.

The Ear

Late in the sixth week and during the seventh week, the basal turn of the cochlea forms. A depression develops between the saccule and the cochlear duct and constricts to form the ductus reuniens (Fig. 38). The maculae differentiate into sensory and supporting cells concurrently with neural differentiation. The cristae ampullaris form. During the seventh week, the stapes ring emerges around the stapedial artery. At the same time, the lamina stapedialis (otic mesenchyme) appears. It will become the footplate and annular ligament. Interhyale cells aggregate as precursors of the stapedius muscle and tendon. Also at about the same time, cartilage is beginning to form in the auricle.

During the eighth week, the first pharyngeal grooves surface and ectoderm thickens and grows as a solid core of epithelium toward the middle ear. The hillocks of His move further apart and begin to develop different shapes that will become portions of the auricle

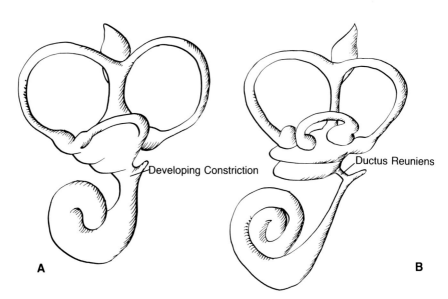

FIG. 38. A: Development of the cochlea and ductus reuniens in the seventh week. **B:** Development of the cochlea and ductus reuniens in the eighth week. (Modified from ref. 63, with permission.)

(Fig. 39). The tympanic ring forms during the ninth week. The malleus and incus are separated and the incudomalleal joint is formed during the eighth week. At 8½ weeks, the incudostapedial joint develops. The interhyale becomes recognizable as the stapedial muscle and tendon. The laterohyale becomes the posterior wall of the middle ear together with the otic capsule, pyramidal process, and part of the facial canal. A portion of the lower part of the facial canal is believed to come from Reichert's cartilage (63). During the eighth week, the semicircular canals and utricle are fully formed. The saccule and endolymphatic duct are formed as well. The sacculo-endolymphatic and utriculo-endolymphatic ducts appear, the stria vascularis begins to develop, and two ridges of cells appear in the cochlea. The inner ridge becomes the spiral limbus, and the smaller outer ridge will become the organ of Corti. Development proceeds from the basal turn to the apical end of the cochlea. The cells that give rise to the tectorial membrane also appear during the eighth week. The precursor of the otic capsule develops further as

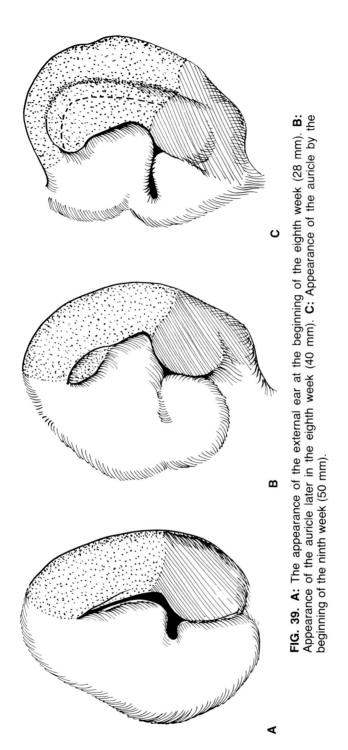

FIG. 39. A: The appearance of the external ear at the beginning of the eighth week (28 mm). **B:** Appearance of the auricle later in the eighth week (40 mm). **C:** Appearance of the auricle by the beginning of the ninth week (50 mm).

precartilage. The lamina stapedialis appears during the eighth week. This will become the vestibular surface of the footplate of the stapes. Rugae appear in the endolymphatic sac. The vestibule begins to develop in the ninth week.

TENTH THROUGH FIFTEENTH WEEK

The Facial Nerve

In the 58- to 80-mm period, extensive branching of the peripheral portions of the facial nerve occurs (Fig. 40). Some divisions reach

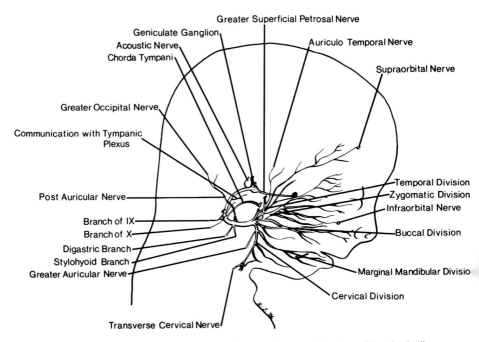

FIG. 40. During the eleventh week (80 mm), extensive branching including communications with other cranial nerves can be seen. The vertical portion of the facial nerve is still anterior with respect to the external auditory meatus (not shown). The vertical portion and main trunk could be injured easily during surgery if the relationship of the auricle to the facial nerve were assumed to be that of an adult. (Modified from ref. 44, with permission.)

the midline. Extensive communication with branches of the trigeminal nerve occurs in the perioral and infraorbital regions. Communications exist between the nervus intermedius and both the eighth nerve and motor root of the seventh nerve. Despite extensive branching of the facial nerve, it begins its vertical course while still in the middle ear, and its relationship to the external and middle ear structures is far more anterior than in the adult (Figs. 41 and 42). In the eleventh week (80 mm), the external petrosal nerve arises from the facial nerve distal to the geniculate ganglion, traveling with a branch of the middle meningeal artery. Branches also arise from the facial nerve between the stapedius and chorda tympani nerves. These branches join together with branches of IX and X to provide sensory innervation to the external auditory canal. Branches to the lateral

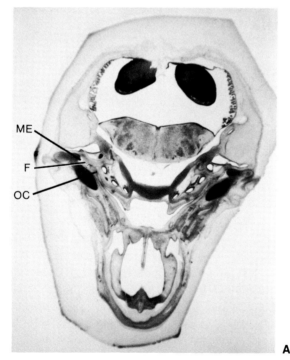

A

FIG. 41. A: Section of a ten-week-old fetus illustrating the facial nerve (F) in contact with otic capsule precartilage (OC), medial to the developing middle ear region (ME). **FIG. 41.** *Continues.*

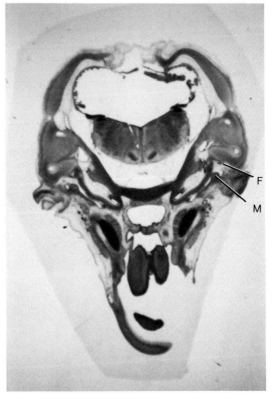

B

FIG. 41. *Continued.* **B:** The facial nerve (F) runs lower in the middle ear than in the adult. The developing Malleus (M) is also seen.

aspects of the eyelids are present, and communication with the zy-gomaticotemporal nerve has begun to develop. Previous communications with branches from cervical nerves have now become communications with the lesser occipital and transverse cervical nerves. The horizontal portion of the facial nerve can be seen distinctly adjacent to the developing otic capsule (Fig. 42B). The nasal muscles are also differentiated at approximately 80 mm.

The relationship between the facial nerve and the parotid gland is about the same at twelve weeks as it was at seven weeks. However, by the time the fetus reaches 80 mm in length, complicated connections between the superficial and deep portions of the parotid primordium can be seen (Fig. 43) (48). At 14 to 15 weeks, the geniculate ganglion is fully developed and facial nerve relationships to

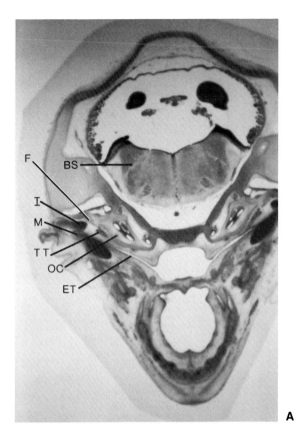

A

FIG. 42. A: In this 10¹/₂-week-old fetus, the horizontal portion of the facial nerve (F) can be seen distinct from the maturing otic capsule precartilage (OC). The malleus (M), incus (I), eustachian tube (ET), tensor tympani (TT), and brain stem (BS) are also seen. **FIG. 42.** *Continues.*

middle ear structures have developed more fully (Figs. 44–47). While the above growth has occurred, the facial nerve has remained in association with the mesenchyme, which differentiates into the labyrinth and mastoid.

The Ear

During the tenth week, pneumatization begins. The stapes changes from its original ring shape to a stirrup shape (Fig. 48). Also during

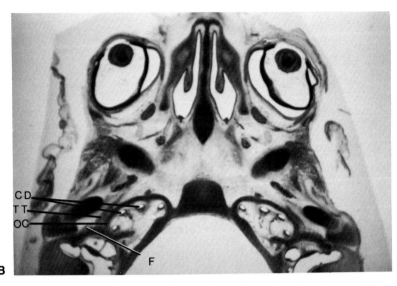

B

FIG. 42. *Continued.* **B:** In a twelve-week-old fetus, the facial nerve (F) is well formed and separate from the developing otic capsule (OC) and turns of the cochlear duct (CD).

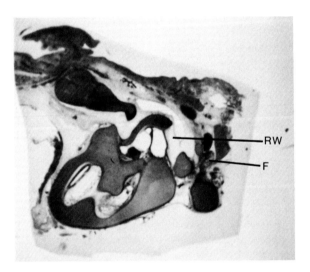

FIG. 43. The right ear of another 14-week-old fetus illustrates the position of the vertical portion of the developing facial nerve (F) at the level of the developing round window niche (RW).

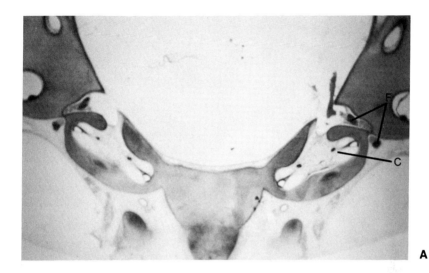

A

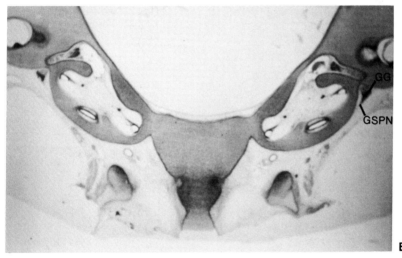

B

FIG. 44. A: In this 14-week-old fetus, portions of the facial nerve (F) can be seen in the internal auditory canal and the middle ear. The developing cochlea (C) is also seen well. **B:** At a slightly lower level, the geniculate ganglion (GG) and greater superficial petrosal nerve (GSPN) can be seen. **FIG. 44.** *Continues.*

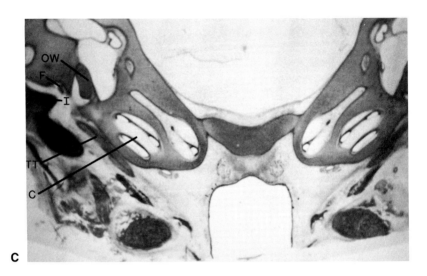

C

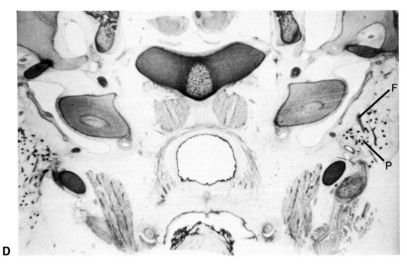

D

FIG. 44. *Continued.* **C:** The horizontal portion of the facial nerve (F) courses above the oval window (OW). The developing tensor tympani (TT) is seen lateral to the cochlea (C). Development of the incus (I) continues as the shape of the ossicles becomes better defined. **D:** Branches of the facial nerve (F) are seen clearly in the parotid primordium (P).

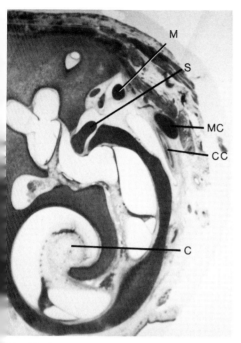

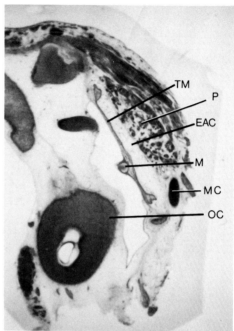

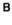

B

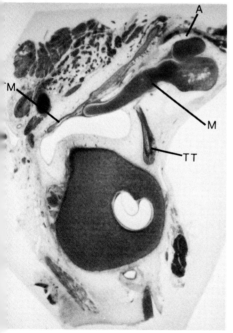

FIG. 45. A: In the left ear of a 14¹/₂-week-old fetus, the stapes (S) and cochlea (C) are visible. The malleus (M) is seen in relation to a portion of Meckel's cartilage (MC) that was formally connected with the malleus. Cartilaginous cells (CC) forming a portion of the annulus of the tympanic membrane are also visible. **B:** In the same fetus, the tympanic membrane (TM) may be seen in conjunction with the malleus handle (M) lateral to the otic capsule (OC), and medial to the region of the future external auditory canal (EAC). A portion of Meckel's cartilage (MC) is also visible adjacent to parotid gland tissue (P). **C:** The right ear of the same fetus shows the malleus (M) in the attic (A) and attaching to the tympanic membrane (TM). The tendon of the tensor tympani (TT) is also visible extending toward the malleus handle.

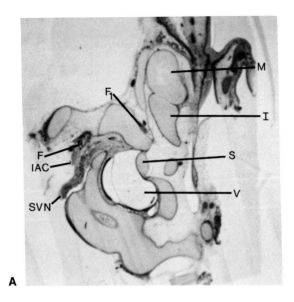

A

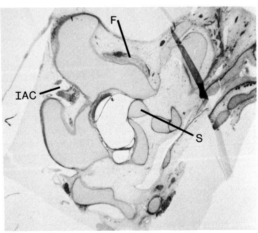

B

FIG. 46. A: In this 15-week-old fetus, the superior vestibular nerve (SVN) and facial nerve (F) can be seen in the internal auditory canal (IAC). The malleus (M), incus (I), stapes (S), and vestibule (V) are also visible. The middle ear is still small, but the ossicles are approaching adult size. A small section of the horizontal position of the facial nerve is visible (F_1). **B:** In a lower section, the area of the second genu of the facial nerve may be seen (F) as the nerve turns posteriorly in the region of the geniculate ganglion. This is often referred to incorrectly as the first genu. The first genu is in the brain stem. The internal auditory canal (IAC) and stapes (S) are labeled for orientation. (Masson trichrome stain.) **FIG. 46.** *Continues.*

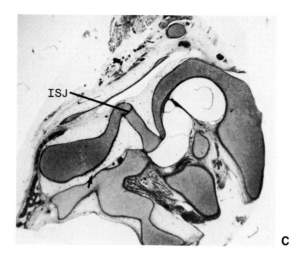

C

FIG. 46. *Continued.* **C:** In the left ear of the same fetus, a well-formed incudostapedial joint can be seen (ISJ). The middle ear is still small, and the space between the incus and the otic capsule (*arrow*) is narrower than in the adult.

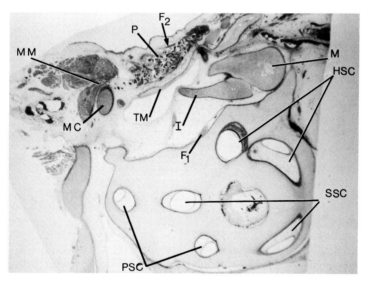

FIG. 47. In the right ear of another 15-week-old fetus, the horizontal (HSC), posterior (PSC), and superior (SSC) semicircular ducts can be seen. The horizontal portion of the facial nerve (F_1) is seen in relationship to the incus (I), malleus (M), and developing tympanic membrane (TM). Lateral to the tympanic membrane, facial nerve branches (F_2) are visible within the parotid gland. The masseter muscle (MM) and a portion of Meckel's cartilage (MC) are also visible.

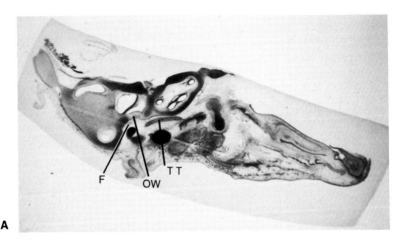

A

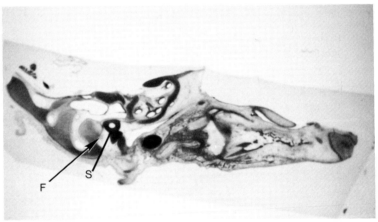

B

FIG. 48. A: The left ear of this 12½-week-old fetus reveals the horizontal portion of the facial nerve (F) coursing near the region of the oval window (OW). Its course superior to the oval window can be seen in a higher section in the same fetus (not shown). The tensor tympani muscle (TT) is also visible. **B:** A slightly lower section of the same fetus reveals the facial nerve (F) and the stapes (S) partially changed from ring to stirrup shape. Ordinarily, this change would be more advanced by 12½ weeks. The fetus illustrated may be somewhat younger than estimated.

the tenth week, the tectorial membrane appears. At about the same time, macular cell types are apparent and the otolithic membrane is being formed. The cupulae appear, and otoconia are first noted. During the eleventh week, the vestibular end-organs are formed. At twelve weeks, the perichondrium of the otic capsule appears. At the same time, the scala tympani develops its space. The scala vestibuli does not develop until the 15th week.

During the eleventh and twelfth weeks, the fissula ante fenestram and fossula post fenestram develop. Both are invaginations of vestibular periotic tissue into the lateral wall of the otic capsule. The fossula post fenestram occurs in only about two-thirds of fetuses. Between the twelfth and 28th weeks, four primary mucosal sacs emerge. The saccus anticus gives rise to the anterior pouch von Tröltsch. The saccus medius gives rise to the epitympanum and petrous area. The saccus superior gives rise to the posterior pouch of von Tröltsch, part of the mastoid, and the inferior incudal space. The saccus posterior gives rise to the round window and oval window niches and the sinus tympani. Also at twelve weeks, fusion of the hillocks to form the auricle is complete. Considerable development of the external ear has occurred by the twelfth week (Fig. 49). By the 15th week, the tympanic ring is almost fully developed. Also in the 15th week, the first of the 14 ossification centers can be identified, the scala vestibuli develops its space, and formation of the membranous labyrinth without the end-organ is complete.

SIXTEENTH WEEK THROUGH BIRTH

The Facial Nerve

Between 16 and 20 weeks, the facial nerve, arterioles, venules, and the stapedius muscle lie in a sulcus on the canalicular wall. The mesenchyme in which they are surrounded is differentiating into connective tissue. Although the middle ear continues to enlarge (Figs. 50 and 51), the facial nerve remains more superficial and anterior in relation to the auricle than in the adult. All definitive communications of the facial nerve are established by the 16th week (146 mm). By 26 weeks ossification has progressed, and growth of

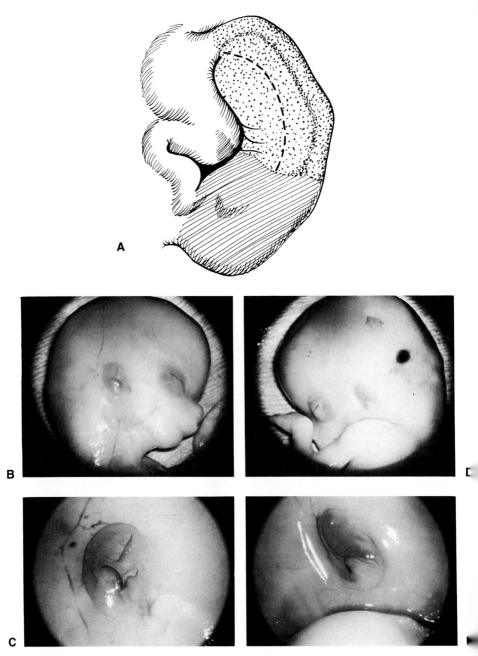

FIG. 49. A: Appearance of the auricle at the beginning of the twelfth week (85 mm). **B:** Right side of the head of a 75-mm fetus (approximately eleven weeks). The photograph was taken prior to dissection. **C:** Close-up of the right ear of the fetus pictured in **B. D:** The left side of the same fetus illustrates asymmetry in development. **E:** A close-up of the left ear shows that auricular development is considerably retarded in comparison with the right side. This appearance is more likely to be seen at around the eighth week.

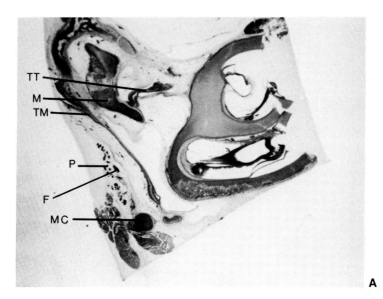

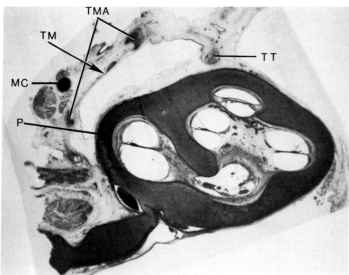

FIG. 50. **A:** In the left ear of this 17-week-old fetus, the facial nerve has already exited the temporal bone to the stylomastoid foramen. The main trunk of the facial nerve (F) can be seen in the parotid gland (P) in relation to a section of Meckel's cartilage. M, malleus. **B:** In the right ear of the same fetus, the tympanic membrane (TM) and developing tympanic membrane annulus (TMA) are visible, along with Meckel's cartilage (MC) and the tensor tympani (TT). The distance between the tympanic membrane and the promontory (P) remains somewhat less than expected in a normal adult ear.

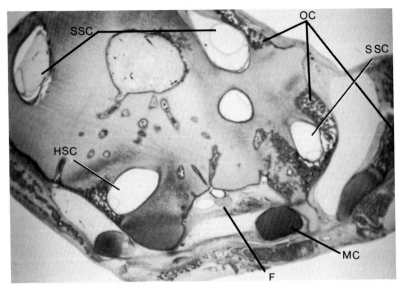

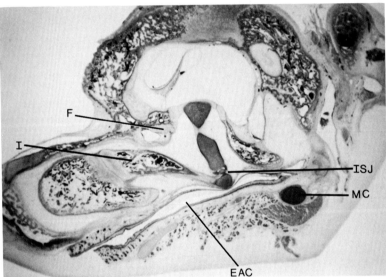

FIG. 51. A: In this 19½-week-old fetus (left ear), the facial nerve (F) can be seen coursing above the oval window (not shown) and lateral to the horizontal semicircular canal (HSC). The superior semicircular canal (SSC) is also seen. Ossification centers (OC) are visible in several areas. **B:** Ossification is also visible on the incus (I), and a well-developed incudostapedial joint (ISJ) is present. The facial nerve (F) can be seen in its horizontal portion. The external auditory canal (EAC) is also seen, as well as Meckel's cartilage (MC). **FIG. 51.** *Continues.*

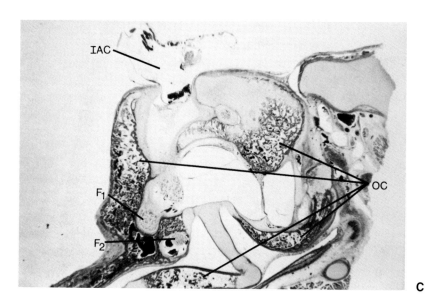

C

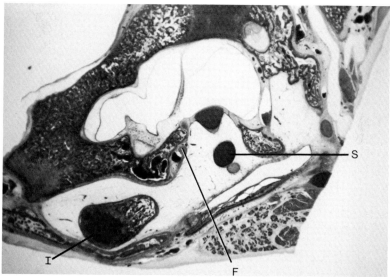

D

FIG. 51. *Continued.* **C:** Masson trichrome staining of the right ear of the same fetus reveals the ossification centers (OC) even more clearly. The internal auditory canal (IAC) is visible. The facial nerve can also be seen in its labyrinthine (F_1) and horizontal (F_2) portions. **D:** Another section of the right ear specimen shows the relationship among the facial nerve (F), the stapes (S), and the incus (I).

the outer layer of periosteal bone has resulted in partial closure of the sulcus into a fallopian canal (Figs. 52–54). The deep surface is completed first. By 35 weeks, a bony ridge has formed to separate the geniculate ganglion from the epitympanic rim. In late fetal life, the facial canal is closed by bone in most cases (Fig. 55) except in the anterior cranial portion where it remains open to form the facial hiatus along the floor of the middle cranial fossa. However, at least 25% of fallopian canals have the dehiscences, with the most common site adjacent to the oval window (69). The dehiscences range from 0.5 mm to the entire horizontal portion, but they are usually no larger than about 2×3 mm in size. This most common area of dehiscence is probably related to the stapedial artery. Some investigators have reported the incidence of dehiscence to be as high as 55% (70) (see Chapter 4).

By the time of birth, the facial nerve has developed into a complex, but generally consistent, structure (Figs. 56–59). Of particular surgical interest is a study by Sammarco et al. (42) on the mandibular ramus in stillborns, in which 17 of 24 facial halves were found to have some or all mandibular branches of the cervical facial ramus below the angle of the mandible. Nineteen of 24 had two or three mandibular branches. All mandibular branches were above the mandibular margin as it crossed the facial artery. In 16, all branches passed over the facial artery and in the rest they straddled the facial artery. At birth, the anatomy of the facial nerve approximates that of the adult except for its exit through the superficially located stylomastoid foramen. Adult anatomy will occur in this region as the mastoid tip develops after birth.

The Ear

The ossicles reach their adult size at 16 weeks. Ossification appears first on the long process of the incus. The head and short process of the incus originate from Meckel's cartilage, and the long process is formed from Reichert's cartilage. The manubrium of the malleus is formed from Reichert's cartilage. The head and neck of the malleus are formed from Meckel's cartilage. The anterior process of the malleus is from the process of Folius (mesenchyme bone)

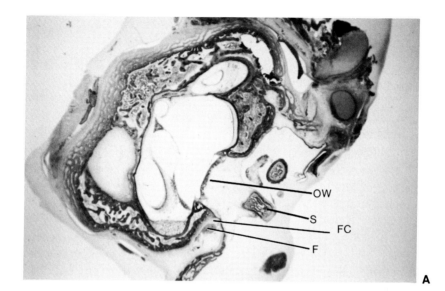

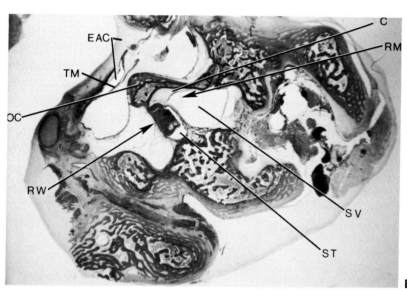

FIG. 52. A: This specimen from an infant born at five months gestation shows the facial nerve (F) in the fallopian canal (FC) posterior to the stapes (S). The oval window (OW) is well formed. The fallopian canal is somewhat more developed than usual. **B:** Even at five months of fetal age, the middle ear space is extremely small and there is little space between the tympanic membrane (TM) and the bony otic capsule (OC). In this section, the external auditory canal (EAC), round window (RW), lateral cochlear wall (C), scala vestibulate (SV), Reissner's membrane (RM), scala media (SM), and scala tympani (ST) are also seen.

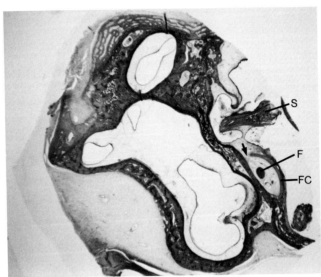

FIG. 53. This 6½-month-old fetus was born prematurely and survived 13 days. A section through the upper portion of the oval window region reveals a portion of the stapes (S) and of an enclosed fallopian canal (FC) containing a section of facial nerve (F). The fallopian canal has a small dehiscence (*arrow*).

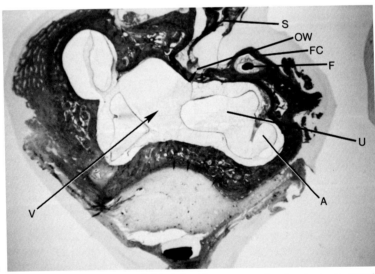

A

FIG. 54. A: The right ear of this infant born prematurely at seven months reveals a well-formed fallopian canal (FC) with a small portion of facial nerve (F) visible. The stapes (S), vestibule (V), utricle (U), oval window region (OW), and a semicircular canal ampulla (A) can be seen as well. **FIG. 54.** *Continues.*

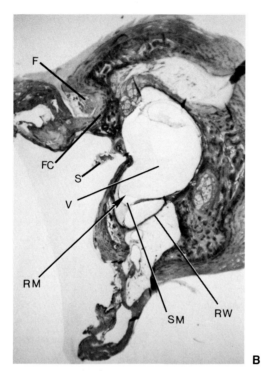

B

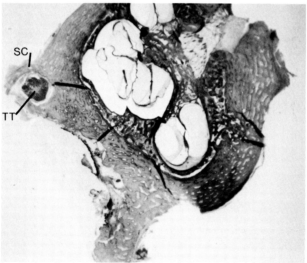

C

FIG. 54. *Continued*. **B:** In the left ear of the same specimen, the fallopian canal (FC) is also formed. The facial nerve (F) is seen within the canal. Portions of the stapes (S), vestibule (V), the round window (RW), and the hook region of the cochlea with Reissner's membrane (RM), the scala media (SM), and scala tympani are visible. **C:** Another section of the same specimen reveals the semicircular canal (SC) containing the tensor tympani muscle (TT).

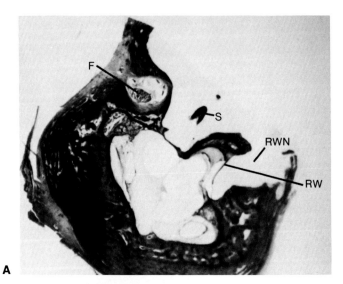

A

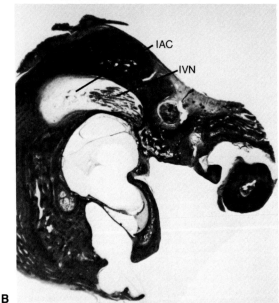

B

FIG. 55. A: The middle ear is excavated and adult relationships are present in this specimen taken from an infant born at eight months' gestation. This section reveals a small segment of the horizontal portion of the facial nerve (F) enclosed in the fallopian canal, the stapes (S), the round window membrane (RW), and the round window niche (RWN). **B:** A lower section also shows the inferior vestibular nerve (IVN) in the internal auditory canal (IAC).

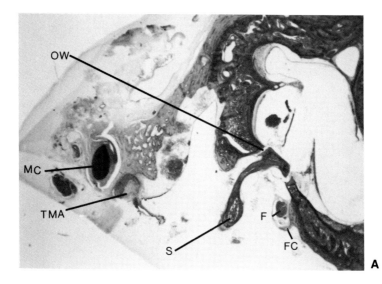

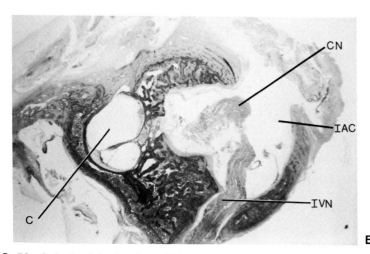

FIG. 56. A: In the fully developed left middle ear of this newborn who died at one hour of age, a remnant of Meckel's cartilage (MC) is still visible near the insertion of the tympanic membrane into its annulus (TMA). The stapes (S) is in the oval window (OW), and the annulus of the footplate has differentiated, separating the footplate from the otic capsule. The horizontal portion of the facial nerve (F) and fallopian canal (FC) are also visible. **B:** Another section of the same specimen shows the basal turn of the cochlea (C), the cochlear nerve (CN), internal auditory canal (IAC), and inferior vestibular nerve (IVN), containing Scarpa's ganglion cells. **FIG. 56.** *Continues.*

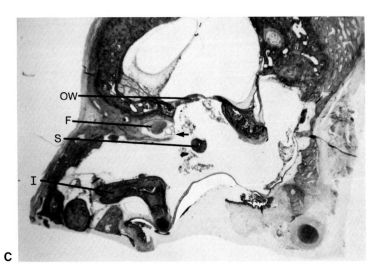

C

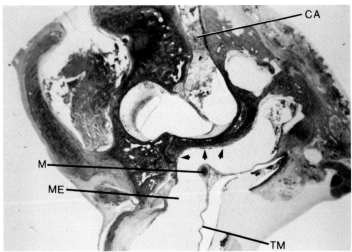

D

FIG. 56. *Continued.* **C:** In the right ear of the same specimen, there is a fallopian canal dehiscence (*arrow*) overlying the oval window (OW). There is soft tissue over the dehiscence, but there is no bone in this region. Portions of the facial nerve (F), stapes (S), and the malleus (M) are visible. **D:** Although fluid is present in the middle ear (ME), a normal amount of space exists between the tympanic membrane (TM) with its incorporated malleus (M), and the medial wall of the middle ear (*arrows*). The cochlea aqueduct (CA) is seen clearly.

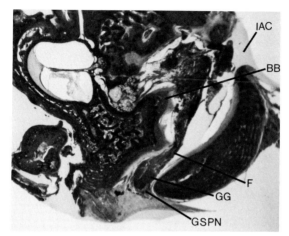

FIG. 57. The left ear of another newborn who died at one hour of age illustrates the full development of the facial nerve (F) as it courses anterior to "Bill's bar" (BB) in the internal auditory canal (IAC). It reaches the geniculate ganglion (GG), and the greater superficial petrosal nerve (GSPN) is given off.

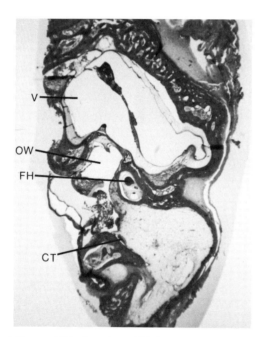

FIG. 58. The left ear of this five-day-old infant highlights the position of the facial nerve in its horizontal (FH) course and a small segment of the chorda tympani nerve (CT) distal to its separation from the vertical portion of the facial nerve (not shown). The oval window region (OW) and vestibule (V) are labeled for orientation.

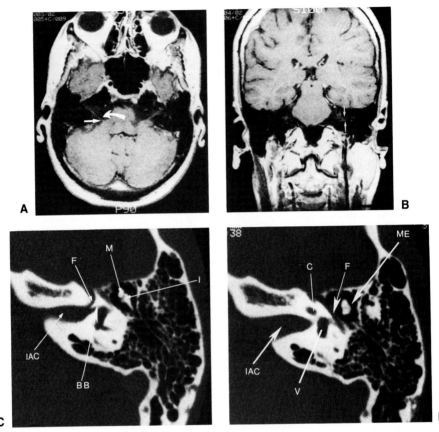

FIG. 59. Computerized tomography (CT) and magnetic resonance imaging (MRI) are now capable of defining facial nerve position in many cases, as illustrated by the following images of normal patients. **A:** An axial MRI showing the acoustic (*straight arrow*) and facial (*curved arrow*) nerves at their junctions with the brain stem. The nerves course toward the internal auditory canal. **B:** A coronal MRI illustrating the seventh and eighth nerve complex in the internal auditory canal (*arrows*). **C:** An axial CT showing the internal auditory canal (IAC), Bill's bar (BB), canal for the labyrinthine portion of the facial nerve (F), malleus (M), and the incus (I). **D:** An axial CT at a lower level illustrating the horizontal portion of the facial nerve (F), the internal auditory canal (IAC), the basal turn of the cochlea (C), the vestibule (V), and the middle ear (ME). **FIG. 59.** *Continues.*

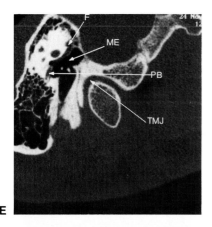
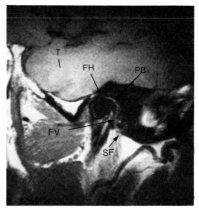

E   G

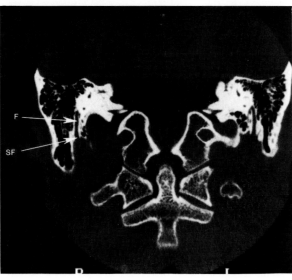

F

FIG. 59. *Continued.* **E:** A sagittal CT in which the horizontal portion of the facial nerve (F) can be seen extending from the region of the geniculate ganglion through the middle ear to the region of the pyramidal bend (PB). The middle ear space (ME) and temporomandibular joint (TMJ) are also visible. **F:** A coronal CT illustrating the vertical portion of the facial nerve canal (F) coursing toward the stylomastoid foramen (SF). **G:** A sagittal MRI that demonstrates the horizontal (FH) and vertical (FV) portions of the facial nerve. The pyramidal bend (PB) and stylomastoid (SF) are clearly visible, as is the temporal lobe (T). (The CT and MRI figures above were produced under the direction of David P. Mayer, M.D., Graduate Imaging Center, Philadelphia, Pennsylvania.)

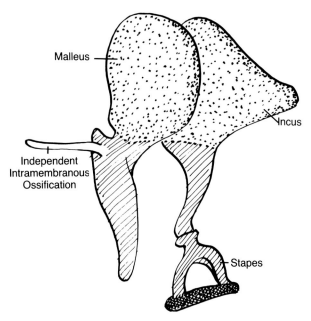

FIG. 60. Current theory of the origin of the ossicles. Stippled areas are derived from Meckel's cartilage, striped areas come from Reichert's cartilage, and the cross-hatched area (vestibular surface) of the footplate is derived from the otic capsule. (Modified from ref. 63, with permission.)

(Fig. 60). By the 17th week, ossification centers become visible on the medial surface of the malleus, spreading to the manubrium and head. Stapes ossification begins at the obturator surface of the stapedial base between 18 and 19 weeks. The cartilaginous vestibular surface of the base is derived from the lamina stapedialis of the otic capsule. The rest of the stapes comes from Reichert's cartilage. This information is different from previous findings. However, it is the currently accepted understanding of ossicular embryology (64).

At 16 weeks, auricular components are recognizable, but they are bulky and not fully formed. At 20 weeks, the auricle has reached its adult shape (Figs. 61 and 62). However, it continues to grow until about the age of nine. The Darwinian tubercle does not usually appear until the sixth month. At 20 weeks, the last of the ossification centers appears. In addition, the stria vascularis and tectorial membrane are completed. At approximately 21 weeks, the epithelial core in the external meatus begins to resorb to form the ear canal (Figs.

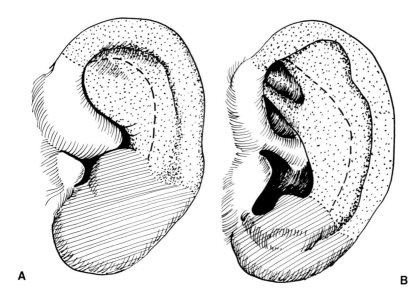

FIG. 61. A: Shape of the auricle at 16 weeks. **B:** Auricular appearance at 20 weeks.

50 and 52). The innermost layer remains as the superficial layer of the tympanic membrane. At around the 22nd week, loose connective tissue extends laterally from the epitympanum between the tympanic process of the squamous bone and the otic capsule forming a tissue space, the future antrum. The air spaces connected with the middle ear expand to form the antrum, epitympanic space, and pneumatized mastoid. This process is not completed until after birth. Ossification of the otic capsule is completed by about the 23rd week. The last area to ossify is the fissula ante fenestra which may remain cartilaginous throughout life.

The membranous and bony labyrinth are adult size by the 23rd week except for the endolymphatic sac. During this period, the two cochlear ridges divide. The inner ridge cells become the spiral limbus. The outer ridge cells become hair cells, pillar cells, Hensen's cells, and Deiters' cells of the organ of Corti. The bony spiral lamina also develops. The inner spiral sulcus, inner and outer tunnels, and basilar membrane develop during the sixth month, as do the tunnel of Corti and the space of Nuel.

Resorption of the ear canal plug is completed at the 28th week,

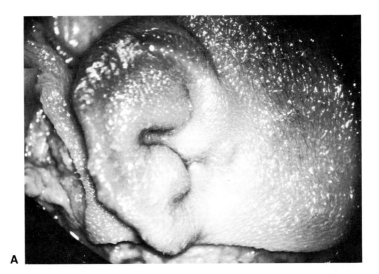

A

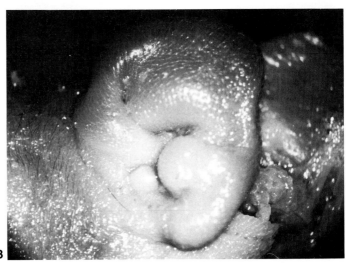

B

FIG. 62. A: Photograph of the right ear of the oldest fetus obtained for dissection in this study. The fetus aborted spontaneously at approximately 20 weeks menstrual age, or 18 weeks fertilization age. Autopsy identified no major anomalies. The right ear shows an identifiable helix, tragus, anti-tragus, lobule, and early development of the antihelix and concha. It is consistent with about 16 weeks of fetal development. Its immaturity may be owing to an incorrect estimate of menstrual age, or to defective development that may have been associated with the spontaneous abortion. **B:** Marked asymmetry is seen when the left ear of the same specimen is examined. The left ear is more consistent with the fetus eleven to twelve weeks old. Both fetuses with marked asymmetry of auricular development examined in this study had culminated in spontaneous abortion for unknown reasons. (Figs. 49B–49E depict the other fetus.)

and the ear canal is open. At the same time, the eardrum appears. The squamous layer is derived from ectoderm. The fibrous layer comes from mesoderm. The mucosal layer is an endoderm derivative. Stapes ossification is complete by the 28th week except for the vestibular surface of the footplate. By the 30th week, excavation of the tympanic cavity is complete. However, the tympanic cavity will remain filled with embryonal connective tissues until after birth.

At birth, the shape of the auricle is the same as in the adult. The ear canal is not ossified. Ossification will be completed at about age three. Full size of both the auricle and ear canal is achieved at about age nine. The middle ear is well formed and enlarges only slightly after birth. It is still partially filled with mucoid connective tissue, which is resorbed within a few months, and pneumatization of the middle ear, antrum, and mastoid continues. Pneumatization of the petrous portion starts last and continues until puberty. The mastoid process appears at about the age of one and is not fully formed until around age three. The developing mastoid tip carries the stylomastoid foramen and the facial nerve medially and inferiorly into their adult positions. The tympanic ring also ossifies at about age three. The eustachian tube is about 17 mm at birth and grows to approximately 36 mm. The malleus, incus, and stapes are of adult size and shape at birth. Part of the manubrium of the malleus remains cartilaginous and never ossifies. The same is true for the vestibular surface of the stapes. The petrous, squamous, and tympanic ring portions of the temporal bone are distinguishable at birth, as is the styloid process. The membranes and bony labyrinth are of adult size at birth except for the endolymphatic sac. This is the first structure to appear and the last to stop growing. It continues to enlarge until adulthood.

REFERENCES

1. Rabl K. Uber das geblet des nervus facialis. *Anat Anz* 1887;2:219–227.
2. Mendel E. Ueber den kernursprung des augen-facialis. *Neurol Centralbl* 1887;23:537–542.
3. Popowsky L. Zur entwicklungsgeschichte des n. facialis beim menschen. *Morphol Jahrb* 1985;23: 329–380.

4. Marinesco G. L'origine du facial superieur. *Rev Neurol (Paris)* 1989;6:30–33.
5. Marinesco G. L'origine du facial superieur. *Ann Med Interne (Paris)* 1989;3: 12–15.
6. Futamura R. Uber die entwickelung der facialismuskalatur des menschen. *Anal Heft* 1906;30:433– 516.
7. Streeter GL. On the development of the membranous labyrinth and the acoustic and facial nerves in the human embryo. *Am J Anat* 1907;6:139–165.
8. Harman NB. The origin of the facial nerve. *Br Med J* 1907;2:1296–1297.
9. Bruce A, Pirie JHH. On the origin of the facial nerve. *Rev Neurol Psychiatr* 1908;6:685–697.
10. Streeter GL. The nuclei of origin of the cranial nerves in the 10 mm human embryo. *Anat Rec* 1908; 2:111–115.
11. Harman NB. On the origin of the facial nerve. *Rev Neurol Psychiatr* 1909;7: 88–92.
12. Sheldon RE. The phylogeny of the facial nerve and chorda tympani. *Anat Rec* 1909;3(12):593–617.
13. Yagita K. Experimentelle untersuchungen uber den ursprung des nervus facialis. *Anat Anz* 1910;37: 195–218.
14. Gregoire R. Le nerf facial et la parotide. *J Anat Physiol* 1912;48:437–447.
15. Papez JW. Subdivisions of the facial nucleus. *J Comp Neurol* 1927;43(1):159–191.
16. Vernon E. The intrapontine part of the motor root of the facial nerve. *J Anat* 1931;66:66–75.
17. Hewer EE. The development of nerve endings in the human foetus. *J Anat* 1935;69:369–374.
18. Okinaka S, Sano T. Extrapyramidaler kern und extrapyramidale faser im facialis. *Ztschr Zellforsch uber Mikr Anat* 1936;25:240–246.
19. Pearson AA. The development of the motor nuclei of the facial nerve in man. *J Comp Neurol* 1946; 85:461–476.
20. Pearson AA. The roots of the facial nerve in human embryos and fetuses. *J Comp Neurol* 1947;87:139–159.
21. Van Campenhout E. Le development du systeme nerveux peripherique cranien chez l'embryon de crocodile. *Assoc Anat* 1953;39(4):402–406.
22. Tamari MJ. The facial nerve. *J International College of Surgeons* 1955;23(3), Pt.1:364–370.
23. Fabiani F. Considerazioni sulla suddivisione del nucleo motore del facciale e del complesso della radiac discendente del trigemino. *Riv Patologia Nervosa Mentale* 1955;76(2):435–460.
24. Fabiani F. L'ontogenesi del nucleo motore del nervo facciale nell'uomo. *Riv Patologia Nervosa Mentale* 1957;78(2):421–471.
25. Batten EH. The behavior of the epibranchial placode of the facial nerve in the sheep. *J Comp Neurol* 1957;108(3):393–419.
26. Batten EH. The origin of the acoustic ganglion in sheep. *J Embryol Exp Morphol* 1958;6:597–615.
27. Revazov BC. Intracerebral pathway of the facial nerve during human intrauterine development. *Arkh Anat Gistol Embriol* 1958;35(5):106–107.
28. Ponomareva IA. The connections of the facial nerve and the trigeminal nerve. From Sbornik trudov, posvyashchennyi 60-letiya so dnya rozhdeniya i 25-letiyu nauchnopedagogicheskoi deyatelnosti v Kazalhstane professora P.O.; Isaeva (Alma-Ata), 1953;136–137.

29. LaVelle A, LaVelle FW. Neuronal reaction to injury during development severance of the facial nerve in utero. *Exp Neurol* 1959;1:82–95.
30. Hahlbrock K. Zweiteilung des n. facialis im Warzenfortsatz. *Arch Ohren usw Heilk u Z Hals-usw Heilk* 1960;174:465–469.
31. Blinkov CM. Nucleus nervi facialis accessorius and interlacing of the fibres of the root of the principal nucleus in man. *Zh Neuropat Psykhiot* 1961;61(2):265–270.
32. Anson BJ, Harper DG, Warpeha RL. Surgical anatomy of the facial canal and facial nerve. *Ann Otol* 1963;72:713–734.
33. Rossberg G. Ohrmissbildungen und contergan. *Z Laryngol Rhinol Otol* 1963;42:473–498.
34. LaVelle A. Mitochondrial changes in developing neurons. *Am J Anat* 1963; 113:175–187.
35. Eyries C, Chouard CH. Les origines reelles du nerf facial. *Ann Otolaryngol (Paris)*, 1963;80(9): 775–802.
36. Samengo LA. Consideraciones embriologicas y anatomoquirurgicas de la parotida. *Rev Assoc Med Argent* 1964;78(9):513–516.
37. Fischer J, Malik V. A histochemical study on the effect of transection of the facialis nerve on the picture of glycerophosphate, lactate, succinate, malate and glutamate dehydrogenase in the cells of the facial nerve nucleus. *Acta Histochem Bd* 1964;19:369–376.
38. Annon BJ. Die embryologie und anatomie des facialiskanals und des facialisnerven. *Arch Ohren Nasen Kehlk* 1965;184(4):269–284.
39. Miehlke A. Anatomy and clinical aspects of the facial nerve. *Arch Otolaryngol* 1965;81:444–445.
40. Orr MF. Development of acoustic ganglia in tissue cultures of embryonic chick otocysts. *Exp Cell Res* 1965;40:68–77.
41. Courville J. The nucleus of the facial nerve; the relation between cellular groups and peripheral branches of the nerve. *Brain Res* 1966;1(4):338–354.
42. Sammarco GJ, Ryan RF, Longenecker CG. Anatomy of the facial nerve in fetuses and stillborn infants. *Plast Reconstr Surg* 1966;37(4):566–574.
43. Gasser RF, Hendrickx AG. The development of the facial nerve in baboon embryos (Papio sp.). *J Comp Neurol* 1967;129:203–218.
44. Gasser RF. The development of the facial nerve in man. *Ann Otol* 1967;76:37–56.
45. Vidic B. The origin and the course of the communicating branch of the facial nerve to the lesser petrosal nerve in man. *Anat Rec* 1968;162:511–516.
46. Rhoton AL, Kobayashi S, Hollinshead WH. Nervus intermedius. *J Neurosurg* 1968;29:609–618.
47. Jacobs MJ. The development of the human motor trigeminal complex and accessory facial nucleus and their topographic relations with the facial and abducens nuclei. *J Comp Neurol* 1970;138(2):161–194.
48. Gasser RF. The early development of the parotid gland around the facial nerve and its branches in man. *Anat Rec* 1970;167:63–78.
49. Johns ME. The salivary glands: anatomy and embryology. *Otolaryngol Clin North Am* 1977;10(2):261–271.
50. Vidic B. The anatomy and development of the facial nerve. *Ear Nose Throat J* 1978; 57(6):236–242.
51. Carlson BM. The development of facial muscles and nerves in relation to the mobius syndrome. *Otolaryngol Head Neck Surg* 1981;89(6):903–906.

52. Ge, Spector GJ. Labyrinthine segment and geniculate ganglion of facial nerve in fetal and adult human temporal bones. *Ann Otol Rhinol Laryngol* 1981;4(pt 2,suppl 85):1–12.

53. Liston SL. The relationship of the facial nerve and first branchial cleft anomalies—embryologic considerations. *Laryngoscope* 1982;92(11):1308–1310.

54. McRae RG, Lee KJ, Goertzen E. First branchial cleft anomalies and the facial nerve. *Otolaryngol Head Neck Surg* 1983;91(2):197–202.

55. Gasser R, May M. Embryonic development of the facial nerve. In: May M, ed. *The facial nerve*. New York: Thieme, 1986;3–20.

56. Schuknecht HF, Gulya AJ. *Anatomy of the temporal bone with surgical implications*. Philadelphia: Lea & Febiger, 1986;235–303.

57. Ariens K, Cornelius U. *The evolution of the nervous system in invertebrates, vertebrates and man*. Haarlem, The Netherlands: De Erven F. Bohn, 1929;78,92–93,106–107,119–122,167.

58. Patten BM. *Human embryology*. Philadelphia: Blakiston, 1946;112–113,306–314,371–375,435.

59. Hamilton WJ, Boyd JD, Mossman HW. *Human embryology*, 2nd ed. Cambridge, Massachusetts: Heffer, 1952;157,277–280, 306, 310.

60. Lawrence M. The double innervation of the tensor tympani. *Ann Otol Rhinol Laryngol* 1962;71:705–718.

61. Bast TH, Anson, BJ. *The temporal bone and the ear*. Springfield, Illinois: Charles C. Thomas, 1949;3–377.

62. Davies J. *Embryology of the head and neck in relation to the practice of otolaryngology*. Rochester, Minnesota: American Academy of Ophthalmology and Otolaryngology, 1957; 35–40.

63. Pearson AA, Jacobson AD. *The development of the ear*. Rochester, Minnesota: American Academy of Ophthalmology and Otolaryngology, 1973; Ch 1,1–50; Ch 2,1–54; Ch 3,1–25.

64. Pearson AA. Developmental anatomy of the ear. In: English GM, ed. *Otolaryngology*, vol 1. Hagerstown, Maryland: Harper and Row, 1987; Ch 1,1–68.

65. Anson BJ. Developmental anatomy of the ear. In: Paparella MM, Shumrick DA. *Otolaryngology*. Philadelphia: WB Saunders, 1973;3–74.

66. Mall FP. On the age of human embryos. *Am J Anat* 1918;23(2):397–422.

67. Streeter GL. Weight, sitting height, head size, foot length, and menstrual age of the human embryo. *Contrib Embryol* 1920;11(55):143–170.

68. Moore KL. *The developing human—clinically oriented embryology*. Philadelphia: WB Saunders, 1982;78,95.

69. Beddard D, Saunders WH. Congenital defects in the fallopian canal. *Laryngoscope*, 1962;72:112–115.

70. Baxter A. Dehiscence of the fallopian canal. *J Laryngol Otol* 1971;85:587–594.

71. Netter FN. *The Ciba collection of medical illustrations, vol 1, The nervous system*. Summit, New Jersey: Ciba, 1972;47.

72. Coker NJ, Fisch U. Disorders of the facial nerve. In: English GM, ed. *Otolaryngology*. Philadelphia: Harper and Row, 1987; Ch 40, 3–4.

73. Fisch U. *Facial nerve surgery*. Amstelveen, The Netherlands: Kugler, 1977; 21.

3

Clinical Application

In patients with congenital malformations it is usually possible to determine the fetal age at which developmental arrest occurred. This allows one to predict the anatomy of the deformed system on the basis of its usual embryologic development. Moreover, if anomalies are also present in other portions of the same organ system or in different organ systems (such as the kidney), they often reflect interference with development at the same time in fetal life. Applying these well-established principles of medical genetics to the ear, if a congenital anomaly of any portion of the ear can be observed visually, radiologically, or surgically, and if the clinician recognizes the fetal age at which normal development ceased in that portion, then the physician should be able to predict the position of the facial nerve. If it is anomalous, its development is most likely to have been interrupted at the same time as development of the ear, particularly in the case of middle ear malformation. To test the validity of such predictions, observations were made on 11 patients with congenitally malformed ears cared for by the author.

CASE 1

Case 1 has been cared for by the author's partner since 1956 when the patient was four weeks old. He had marked malformation of his right auricle with only a portion of his lobule and helix developed. His external auditory canal was absent. Surgical reconstruction of his auricle was begun in 1961. Unfortunately, no preoperative pictures are available. Figure 1A shows the appearance of his auricle

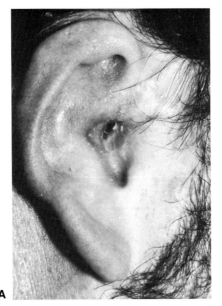
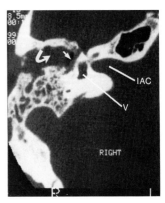

A   **B**

FIG. 1. Case 1. **A:** Appearance of the auricle following numerous otoplasty procedures and prior to surgery by the author. Surgical reconstruction makes it difficult to estimate accurately the fetal age at which the malformation occurred. However, there is essentially no lobule, although there is a good attachment between the face and the portion of the auricle where the lobule should form. The area of the lobule courses superiorly. The position of postauricular surgical scars does not suggest the lobule was rotated superiorly surgically. The junction of the helix and cranium is formed, but most of the helix was obviously absent. The tragus is rudimentary. These features suggest that developmental arrest occurred at about the eighth week of fetal life. **B:** The horizontal portion of the facial nerve (*arrow*) lateral to the vestibule (V) and internal auditory canal (IAC). Scar is present filling the external auditory canal created by previous surgery (*curved arrow*).

after numerous surgical procedures. Previous surgery and radiologic studies reveal that his middle ear was hypoplastic and that his ossicles were rudimentary and fused (Figure 1B).

Analysis

Failure of resolution of the epithelial core to form the ear canal is only helpful in placing the malformation at earlier than 21 weeks.

However, the appearance of the auricle indicates developmental arrest at approximately the beginning of the eighth week. Malformation and fusion of the malleus head and incus body also indicate that the defect occurred late in the seventh week or early in the eighth week. At this time, the middle ear is small and incompletely excavated. The horizontal portion of the facial nerve is above the oval window, but the vertical portion courses more anteriorly and superficially than in the fully developed ear (see Chapter 2, Fig. 35).

Surgical Findings

The patient's most recent operation was performed by the author in 1986 for staged reconstruction of his middle ear for hearing improvement. His middle ear was hypoplastic and appeared anteriorly and inferiorly displaced. He had a monopolar stapes that had been mobilized in 1968 and was still mobile. A rudimentary malleus head and incus body mass was present. The long process of the incus was well formed. The facial nerve was in normal position with respect to the oval window, but it was low and anterior in the surgical field with regard to the expected position of the tympanic membrane. This is usually the case when the middle ear is hypoplastic. The vertical portion coursed considerably more anteriorly and superficially than normal.

Discussion

Recognizing that the anomalies of the auricle, middle ear space, and ossicles head occurred at approximately eight weeks fertilization age allowed accurate prediction of the position of the facial nerve.

CASE 2

Case 2 is a six-year-old who has been followed by the author since the age of three months. His auricle was malformed, with

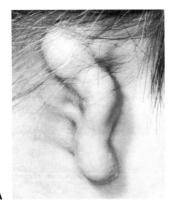 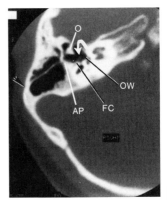

A   **B**

FIG. 2. Case 2. **A:** Appearance of the auricle prior to otoplasty. **B:** CT scan revealing absence of the external auditory canal (*arrow*), an atresia plate (AP) at the level where the tympanic membrane should be, and the ossicular mass (O). The dehiscent horizontal portion of the facial nerve (*curved white arrow*) is seen coursing above the oval window (OW) and entering the fallopian canal (FC) at the pyramidal bend.

portions of the helix, lobule, and tragus recognizable (Fig. 2A). Computed tomography (CT) revealed absence of the external auditory canal and presence of a small middle ear space with an ossicular mass (Fig. 2B).

Analysis

The appearance of the auricle placed the defect at around the eighth week (see Chapter 2, Figs. 39B and 49). By that point, facial nerve development is between that shown in Fig. 35 and that in Fig. 40 in Chapter 2, and the relationship of the nerve to middle ear structures has been established. However, because the middle ear is small and not fully formed, the middle ear and vertical portion of the facial nerve appear anteriorly and inferiorly displaced to the surgeon. Moreover, the vertical portion of the nerve courses more superficially than in the normal adult. This results in the facial nerve coursing through the region where the new ear canal will be constructed.

Surgical Findings

After creating an ear canal and removing the atresia plate, moderately malformed ossicles were identified. The malleus and incus were fused, but an incudomalleal joint could be identified. The stapes was fully developed but immobile. It mobilized easily. The horizontal portion of the facial nerve was in normal position relative to the stapes but dehiscent; the vertical portion of the facial nerve was normal in relation to the middle ear structures. As predicted, the facial nerve and middle ear were more anterior than in a fully developed ear, and the facial nerve coursed anteriorly and laterally more abruptly distal to the pyramidal bend.

Discussion

If the surgeon were to use adult relationships to gauge the position of the middle ear with respect to the position of the external meatus, his entry into the middle ear and mastoid region would be posterior to the vertical portion of the facial nerve and hypoplastic middle ear. Exploration from the point of entry forward would put the facial nerve at risk of injury, especially in light of its abruptly superficial course from the pyramidal bend to the stylomastoid foramen. Its location can be easily and accurately predicted through understanding of its embryology.

CASE 3

Case 3 is a five-year-old female whose hearing loss was noted at age two weeks. Her auricles appeared normal (Fig. 3A). She had complete absence of her right external auditory canal and a 1-mm opening where her left external auditory canal should have been. CT of the left ear revealed bony atresia with an atresia plate, and malleus head and incus body with a well-developed joint (Fig. 3B). CT scan showed that the right middle ear space was smaller, the ossicular mass was more poorly formed and the stapes crura were well developed (Fig. 3C).

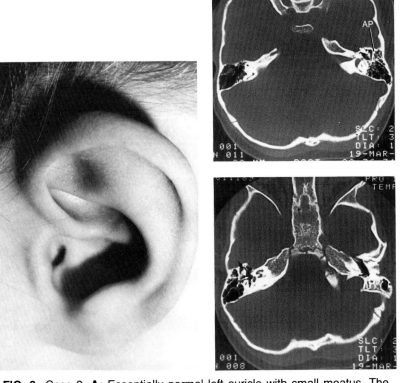

FIG. 3. Case 3. **A:** Essentially normal left auricle with small meatus. The appearance of the right auricle was similar. **B:** CT scan of the left ear showing bony atresia with an atresia plate (AP), and malleus head and incus body with a well-developed joint (*white arrow*). **C:** Right ear illustrating that the middle ear space was smaller, the ossicular mass was more poorly formed (*arrow*), and the stapes crura (*white arrow*) were well formed.

Analysis

Left Ear

On the left, the external auditory canal defect occurred at slightly more than 21 weeks. Epithelial resorption had started, but only to a limited degree. Radiologically, the ossicles of the left ear appeared to be of nearly normal size, but slightly misshapen. The abnormality was limited to the external auditory canal during the fifth month of development, and to the malleus head and incus body. The middle ear was nearly normal in size, and there was no evidence of anomalous development elsewhere. Therefore, it was predicted that the facial nerve would be in normal position.

Right Ear

The canal defect in the right ear happened prior to 21 weeks as there was no evidence of epithelial core resorption. The normal auricle also suggested the absence of major problems in the external ear prior to 20 weeks. However, the middle ear was hypoplastic, and the ossicular defect was considerably worse than on the left. Growth appeared to have stopped early in the eighth week. The portions of the ossicles contributed by Reichert's cartilage were normal (see Chapter 2, Fig. 60). This suggests anterior displacement of the facial nerve with a sharply superficial course in the vertical segment.

Surgical Findings

Left Ear

Surgery was performed upon the left ear in 1986. After removing the atresia plate and creating an external auditory canal, a somewhat bulky, malformed malleus and incus were identified. The long process of the incus was normal. The malleus and the incus were attached with a flexible joint. There was also a normal incudostapedial joint. The stapes was fixed, but its shape was normal. The course of the facial nerve was normal.

Right Ear

Surgery was performed on the right ear in 1987. The middle ear was smaller and more shallow than on the left. Although the stapes and long process of the incus were normal, the head of the malleus and body of the incus were a fused mass. As expected, the nerve and middle ear were more anterior than normal, the horizontal portion of the facial nerve appeared normal in relation to the oval window, but the vertical portion was far anterior in the surgical field. Moreover, because of its rapid lateral course from the pyramidal bend, it had to be skeletonized and used as the posterior limit for the surgically created external auditory canal. Its anterior placement restricted the size of the canal.

Discussion

Differences among the two ears in the fetal age at which the anomalies occurred led to the correct prediction that the facial nerves would be in different positions. If surgical experience on the patient's left ear had been used as a guide to reconstruction on the right ear, the facial nerve could easily have been injured during excision of the atresia plate.

CASE 4

Case 4 is a 50-year-old female born with bilateral complete external auditory canal atresia. She was seen initially in 1987, having had four operations on her left ear and three on her right. She complained of persistent problems with canal stenosis. She has a bilateral mixed hearing loss with a 40 to 50 dB conductive component on the right and a maximal conductive hearing loss on the left. She was able to wear a hearing aid in the right ear, but the left ear canal was closed and too shallow to permit placement of a mold. Her auricles were normal. On the right she had a patent, surgically created external auditory canal and mobile tympanic membrane graft. The left ear canal was closed completely at the level of the meatus. Normal mastoid tips were palpable. CT scan revealed that her middle ear spaces were slightly smaller than usual. Her ossicles were deformed but present. The incudomalleal joint was well developed, and the horizontal portion of the facial nerve was in normal position (Fig. 4). The long process of the incus and the stapes appeared normal (not shown).

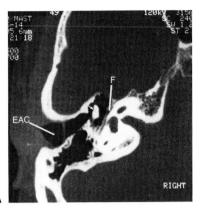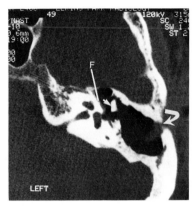

FIG. 4. Case 4. **A:** CT of the right ear showing the horizontal portion of the facial nerve in the fallopian canal (F). An ossicular mass with its incudomalleal joint (*arrows*) and the surgically created external auditory canal (EAC), which is stenotic medially, are also illustrated. **B:** Left ear showing the horizontal portion of the facial nerve (F), malformed ossicles with an incudomalleal joint (*arrow*), and complete obstruction of the external auditory meatus (*curved arrows*).

Analysis

This defect appears limited to the external auditory canals and portions of the ossicles contributed by Meckel's cartilage (see Chapter 2, Fig. 60). Ossicular development indicates that it occurred between 12 and 16 weeks. If a facial nerve abnormality were present, we would expect it to be merely an anterior and superficial course of the vertical segment, less severe than discussed in previous cases. However, the middle ear, portions of the ossicles derived from Reichert's cartilage, otic capsule, and mastoid are reasonably well developed, and the middle ear is not markedly hypoplastic. Therefore, we would expect the facial nerve to be in normal or nearly normal position.

Surgical Findings

Surgery was performed on the left ear to create an ear canal to permit use of a hearing aid. The malleus and incus were malformed and fused, but the joint was clearly present. The long process of the incus and stapes were normal except for stapes fixation. Stapes mobilization was accomplished easily. The course of the facial nerve was normal.

Discussion

Recognizing that the anomaly occurred late and was limited to Meckel's cartilage derivatives allowed accurate prediction of a normal facial nerve course.

CASE 5

Case 5 is a 33-year-old female with left external auditory canal stenosis and conductive hearing loss. She had reportedly undergone an abbreviated exploration of her ear in 1976. She was seen for staged reconstruction initially to permit use of a hearing aid, and eventually to improve hearing. CT scan revealed the middle ear to be only mildly hypoplastic, the mastoid was well formed, and the facial nerves were easily visualized (Fig. 5). The malleus head and incus body were rudimentary, fused, and no incudomalleal joint

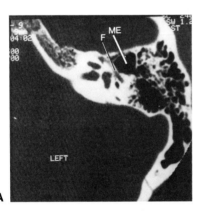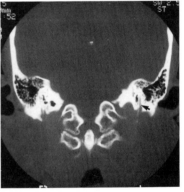

FIG. 5. Case 5. **A:** Axial CT scan revealing a mildly hypoplastic middle ear (ME) and the horizontal portion of the facial nerve in normal position (F). **B:** The vertical portion of the facial nerve also appears normal (*arrow*).

could be ·visualized (not shown). Good mastoid tip development was present.

Analysis

The defect is limited to the external auditory canal and portions of the ossicles derived from Meckel's cartilage (see Chapter 2, Fig. 60). Other otologic structures appear normal. The abnormal ossicular development occurred during the seventh week. Abnormal canal development occurred at around the 28th week, as the ear canal was open but incompletely widened. The facial nerve would be expected to lie in normal or nearly normal position because middle ear excavation and medial ossicular structures are not significantly abnormal.

Surgical Findings

The first stage of reconstruction included canaloplasty, tympanoplasty, stapes mobilization, and resection of a fused incus-malleus mass. It was malformed, and the incudomalleal joint had not developed. The stapes was normal, and middle ear size was at the lower end of normal. The facial nerve was in normal position.

Discussion

Recognition that abnormalities were limited primarily to ossicular derivatives of Meckel's cartilage and the external auditory canal allowed accurate prediction that the facial nerve would be normal. CT scan was also helpful in this case.

CASE 6

Case 6 is a 55-year-old male with bilateral marked canal stenosis, conductive hearing loss, and normal ossicles. He also complained of recurrent ear infections. These infections and the canal stenosis made hearing aid use difficult. CT revealed that his stenotic canal was associated with a moderately hypoplastic middle ear space (Fig. 6).

Analysis

This patient's defect occurred at around the 28th week. The ear canal was open but incompletely widened. Middle ear excavation was also incomplete. These findings suggest fully formed ossicles, possibly with stapes fixation and normal facial nerve position. However, the mildly hypoplastic middle ear suggests that migration may have been incomplete and the vertical portion of the facial nerve may lie more anterior than normal with respect to the ear canal.

Surgical Findings

After elevating a tympanomeatal flap, the vertical portion of the facial nerve was observed anterior to the posterior margin of the bony external auditory canal. As the flap was elevated, the facial

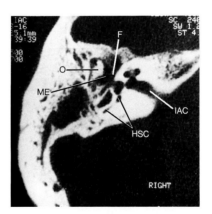

FIG. 6. Case 6. CT shows a moderately hypoplastic, contracted middle ear space (ME). The ossicular heads (O) are crowded in the epitympanum, but they appear fully developed. The horizontal portion of the facial nerve (F) runs in normal relationship to the inner ear structures. The horizontal semicircular (HSC) and internal auditory canal (IAC) are also visualized.

nerve was in the middle of the surgical field. As expected, the hypoplastic middle ear showed stapes fixation. The malleus and incus were also fixed by bony contact with the lateral wall of the epitympanum. The pyramidal process and vertical portion of the facial nerve were well developed and in normal relation to the middle ear structures. The mastoid tip was present, and the distal course of the vertical portion of the facial nerve appeared to be normal.

Discussion

Recognizing that both canal development and middle ear excavation stopped at around the 28th week allowed prediction that the vertical portion of the facial nerve would be nearly normal but would appear anteriorly displaced with respect to the ear canal. This is a particularly hazardous situation, especially when the middle ear space is shallow. In this setting, the facial nerve may be injured with the tip of a pick or elevator while the ear drum is being reflected forward. Usually, only the promontory is medial to the surgical field. In this case, the vertical portion of the facial nerve ran medial to the posterior third of the tympanic membrane.

CASE 7

Case 7 is a 20-year-old female who was cared for from 1957 until 1980 by the author's partner. She was born with markedly stenotic ear canals, but 2- to 3-mm openings were present rather than total atresia. Her first operation by the author was performed in 1982 on her left ear. Radiographs taken at that time are not of satisfactory quality for publication, so her findings are illustrated through CT performed after her surgery was completed (Fig. 7). Radiographs revealed an extremely hypoplastic middle ear space and rudimentary ossicular mass in the left ear, but the stapes was not severely malformed. In the right ear, malformation of the malleus and incus was even more severe, and the stapes could not be visualized. The right ear canal was more stenotic than the left, and a nearly complete atresia plate was present. The middle ear was also more hypoplastic than on the left side.

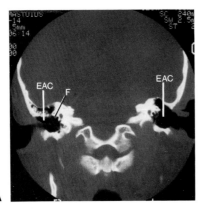
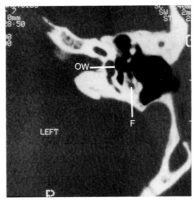

A   B

FIG. 7. Case 7. **A:** Coronal CT scan revealing the widely patent external auditory canal (EAC) on the left. The canal on the right is equally patent, although the angle of the CT scan gives a false impression of soft tissue obstruction. The small, dehiscent facial nerve can be seen on the right (F). **B:** CT of the left ear showing the position of the vertical portion of the facial nerve (F) immediately distal to the pyramidal bend. It is within the newly created external auditory canal and courses even more anteriorly in its distal segment. The oval window (OW) is also visualized. **FIG. 7.** *Continues.*

Analysis

Left Ear

The ossicular defect and middle ear hypoplasia place developmental arrest late in the seventh week. The horizontal portion of the facial nerve should be formed, but the vertical portion of the facial nerve should be more anterior and superficial than normal (see Chapter 2, Fig. 31). The external auditory canal defect appears to have occurred at around 28 weeks.

Right Ear

More severe ossicular malformation and middle ear hypoplasia date this defect at the sixth to early seventh week. Although the facial nerve should course in the region of the oval window, its vertical portion should be considerably more anterior and superficial

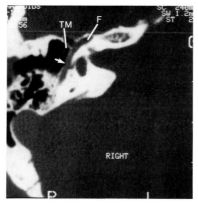

FIG. 7. *Continued.* **C:** The middle ear on the right shows the horizontal portion of the facial nerve (F) with an area of obvious dehiscence (*arrow*). The nerve was partially dehiscent throughout its horizontal course. The relatively narrow ear canal was necessitated by the anterior position of the distal portion of the facial nerve that approached to within 5 mm of the temporomandibular joint (not illustrated). The tympanic membrane (TM) is also visible.

than normal (see Chapter 2, Fig. 23). Canal resorption was substantially incomplete and an atresia plate persisted. This defect probably occurred at around the 24th to 26th week.

Surgical Findings

Left Ear

After creating a large external auditory canal, an extremely shallow middle ear space, rudimentary malleus, and short, deformed incus were found. The stapes was of normal shape and size. The horizontal portion of the facial nerve had areas of dehiscence throughout its course, but its relationship to middle ear structures was normal. The superior aspect of the vertical portion was somewhat anterior to the area where the ear canal should have been. As it coursed distally the nerve became even more abnormally anterior, and the slope of its course from medial to lateral was substantially steeper than normal.

Right Ear

The ear canal was more stenotic than on the left side, and it had a nearly complete atresia plate. The malleus and incus were markedly malformed, appearing as an amorphous mass. There were only nubbins of tissue where the stapes crura should have been. There was no mobile footplate. The facial nerve was dehiscent throughout its horizontal portion and was smaller and more anterior and inferior than on the left side. As expected, the vertical portion of the facial nerve was 3 to 4 mm more anterior than in the more developed left ear. It coursed through the area where the ear canal should have been, and moved almost directly laterally from the pyramidal bend to the anteriorly located stylomastoid foramen. In this region, it coursed only 5 mm posterior to the skeletonized temporomandibular joint in the lower portion of the surgically created ear canal. The facial nerve was skeletonized to maximize ear canal diameter and was visible through bone in the ear canal at the conclusion of the procedure.

Reconstruction resulted in hearing improvement to the 30 dB level on the left and widely patent ear canals permitting use of in-the-ear hearing aids bilaterally.

Discussion

Dates established through the appearance of the ossicles predicted accurately the relatively anterior course of the facial nerve on the left and the markedly abnormal course of the facial nerve on the right. If surgical experience on the left ear had been used as a guide to surgery on the right ear, the facial nerve could easily have been transected while the canal was being widened (Fig. 7A).

CASE 8

Case 8 is a 33-year-old male born with a small, malformed auricle and absent external auditory canal. He underwent otoplastic surgery between 1966 and 1968 (Fig. 8A). Because of previous surgery and the absence of pictures from childhood, the initial

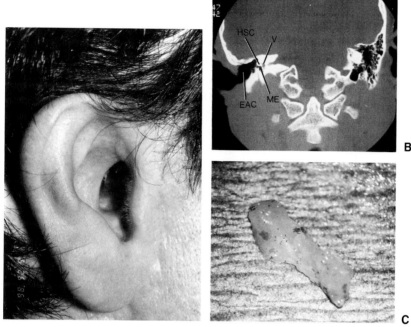

FIG. 8. Case 8. **A:** Because of numerous previous surgical procedures, it is difficult to assess the fetal age at which the auricular deformity occurred. The auricle is small compared with the normal left side. The well-formed lobule and good definition of the helix suggest that developmental arrest probably did not occur until the eleventh or twelfth week. Auricular development is more advanced than middle ear development in this case. **B:** CT scan prior to fenestration showing the vestibule (V), horizontal semicircular canal (HSC), contracted middle ear space (ME), and external auditory canal (EAC). Note that the horizontal semicircular canal lies where the middle ear should be in relation to the external auditory meatus. **C:** Resection of rudimentary ossicular mass. The malleus and incus cannot be identified individually, but their blastomas can be recognized as somewhat more advanced than those shown in Fig. 26 in Chapter 2.

appearance of the auricle could not be determined. Radiologic studies revealed a small middle ear cavity and indistinct ossicular mass. No stapes superstructure or oval window could be identified. Radiographs from that time are of inadequate quality for publication, but Fig. 8B shows the appearance of his ear after creation of an external auditory canal and before a fenestration operation was performed.

Analysis

It is difficult to assess the time of interruption of auricular development with certainty, but the presence of a recognizable portion of helix at its junction with the cranium and the well-formed inferior attachment with absence of a true lobule suggests that the defect occurred around the eighth week (see Chapter 2, Figs. 39A and 39B). However, the markedly malformed ossicles and hypoplastic middle ear place the malformation in this area in the six to seven week period. The horizontal portion of the nerve is low in the middle ear at this time and may overlie the oval window region or promontory. The vertical portion should be present but should course almost directly anteriorly and laterally from the region where the oval window should form (see Chapter 2, Figs. 23 and 30).

Surgical Findings

The author first operated on this patient in 1983. The patient had a tiny middle ear cavity that was anteriorly and inferiorly displaced. The incus-malleus mass was rudimentary without recognizable shapes or an incudomalleal joint (Fig. 8C). The stapes superstructure and oval window were absent. The facial nerve was dehiscent and coursed directly across the promontory. Its position prohibited hearing restoration except through fenestration surgery. Surgery resulted in a dry ear that gave no problems during swimming, and the patient was able to wear a hearing aid. However, for personal and business reasons, he required better directional hearing without amplification. Therefore, a fenestration operation for hearing improvement was performed successfully in 1987.

Discussion

Placing the middle ear and ossicular defect in the six to seven week range allowed accurate prediction of the course of the facial nerve. This was particularly helpful as the nerve was dehiscent except in its distal intratemporal course, so preoperative radiological localization was not possible.

CASE 9

Case 9 is a six-year-old male who has been cared for by the author since the age of five weeks. His right auricle was malformed (Fig. 9A). It had a rudimentary helix and lobule, and a preauricular pit that drained periodically. His left ear was normal (Fig. 9B). CT revealed atresia of the external auditory canal with mild to moderate middle ear hypoplasia (Fig. 9C). The malleus and incus were smaller than on the left, but the incudomalleal joint was present. The long process of the incus and the stapes could not be visualized well. The horizontal fallopian canal was not seen. The inner ear structures were normal.

Analysis

Auricular development appears to have stopped at eight to nine weeks. The presence of an incudomalleal joint also indicated that the fetus must have reached its eighth week before ossicular development was disturbed. This timing is also consistent with the small size of the ossicles and middle ear, and the absence of the external auditory canal. At this time, the facial nerve is expected to be lower and more anterior than usual, and more superficial. The position should be between that seen in Fig. 35 and that illustrated in Fig. 40 in Chapter 2. Inability to visualize the long process of the incus and the stapes may be owing to radiologic technique, but a Reichert's cartilage defect must also be considered, and this suggests an increased chance of partial fallopian canal dehiscence.

Surgical Findings

The first stage of reconstruction was performed when the patient was five years old. The mastoid tip was only partially formed. There was a complete atresia plate between the mastoid tip and the zygomatic arch, and the area in which the bony ear canal had to be created was approximately 5 mm inferior and posterior to the malformed lobule. After a complete mastoidectomy was performed and the atresia plate was removed, the hypoplastic middle ear space was

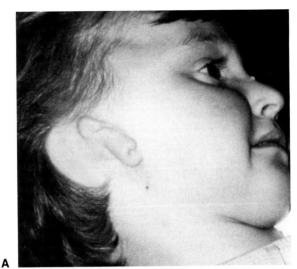

A

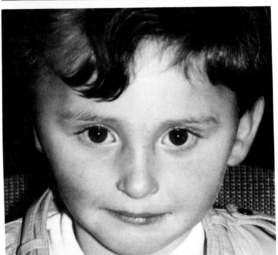

B

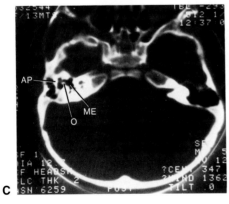

C

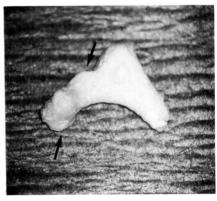

entered. The malleus head and incus body were small but nearly normal in shape. The malleus handle was short. The long process of the incus was also short (Fig. 9D). The stapes was malformed with rudimentary crura, and the footplate was fixed posteriorly but mobile anteriorly. The horizontal portion of the facial nerve was superior to the oval window. The facial nerve was dehiscent on the undersurface of the horizontal portion. However, both structures were more inferiorly and anteriorly placed than normal. The vertical portion of the facial nerve was abnormally anterior and lateral. It was skeletonized and formed the posterior limit of the surgically created external auditory canal. Because of its anterior placement, there was just enough room between the facial nerve and the temporomandibular joint to permit creation of an adequate external auditory canal.

Discussion

Predictions based on embryologic dating were confirmed at the time of surgery. As expected, in the eighth to ninth week an incudomalleal joint was present and the incus body and malleus head were reasonably well formed. The defects in derivatives of Reichert's cartilage are also typical of the eight to nine week time period. The long process of the incus had begun to form but had not reached adult size or shape. The stapes crura were also present but were malformed and had not completed their metamorphosis from ring shape to stirrup shape. The facial nerve dehiscence was coincidental, as it did not occur in an area of the fallopian canal believed to be derived from Reichert's cartilage.

FIG. 9. Case 9. **A:** Appearance of the malformed auricle. **B:** The left auricle is normal, and the right helical-cranial junction is slightly low. **C:** The middle ear is hypoplastic (ME). The ossicular heads (O) are small, and a thick atresia plate is present (AP). **D:** Extraction of malformed incus. Note the short, malformed long process (*arrow*). The incus was removed because it was too far anterior to be useful *in situ* for hearing reconstruction in this hypoplastic middle ear.

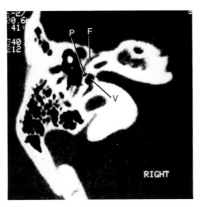 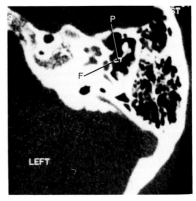

A   B

FIG. 10. Case 10. **A:** The right ear, illustrating the dehiscent horizontal portion of the facial nerve (F) and the tip of the prosthesis (P) entering the vestibule (V) through a surgically-created fenestra. The prosthesis is angled from below the facial nerve superiorly into the vestibular fenestra. **B:** The left ear, showing a portion of the prosthesis (P) adjacent to the dehiscent horizontal portion of the facial nerve (F). **FIG. 10.** *Continues.*

CASE 10

Case 10 is a 20-year-old female with normal external auditory canals and auricles. She had maximal bilateral conductive hearing loss since birth. Radiographs taken prior to her initial surgery were of poor quality. Postoperative CT scans are included to illustrate the findings (Fig. 10).

Analysis

Studies showed no evidence of the long process of the incus, the stapes, or the oval window bilaterally. This Reichert's cartilage defect around the seventh week suggests that the horizontal portion of the facial nerve may be low, and that the fallopian canal may be incomplete.

Surgical Findings

When the patient was 20 years old, right tympanotomy revealed anomalous shortening of the long process of her incus. Although a

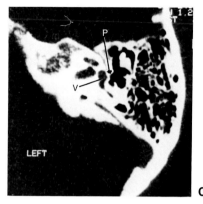

C

FIG. 10. *Continued.* **C:** A higher section showing the tip of the prosthesis (P) entering the vestibule (V) through a surgically-created fenestra just above the malpositioned facial nerve (not shown). There is no evidence of an oval window.

lenticular process appeared to be present, the incus did not reach the area of the footplate. There were only threadlike rudimentary stapes crura, and these were adherent to the dehiscent facial nerve. The facial nerve lay across the area where the oval window should have been. Gentle exploration under the facial nerve revealed no evidence of footplate differentiation. The vertical portion of the facial nerve was also dehiscent and coursed across the posterior aspect of the promontory. It was well anterior to the posterior rim of the ear canal placing it in the middle of the surgical field. Hearing was restored by drilling a small fenestra into the promontory just below the horizontal portion of the facial nerve, and using an incus replacement prosthesis (Fig. 10A). A similar procedure was performed for her left ear approximately one year later. The findings were the same. However, the facial nerve was displaced even more inferiorly. Consequently, the fenestra was drilled just above the facial nerve, rather than below it (Figs. 10B and 10C).

Discussion

This patient's defect in Reichert's cartilage occurred late in the sixth or early in the seventh week prior to formation of the stapes ring. The position of her facial nerve is consistent with that predicted by Fig. 31 in Chapter 2, except that the distal segment of the vertical portion does not turn anteriorly or laterally so abruptly as might be predicted. This maturation is probably associated with more advanced development of the mastoid, which proceeded despite developmental arrest in the derivatives of Reichert's cartilage.

CASE 11

Case 11 is a female who has been cared for by the author's partner since the age of ten days (1956). At that time, she required repair for bilateral choanal atresia. She had narrow external auditory canals bilaterally with normal auricles. Her left ear was operated upon for the first time in 1964. She had a monopolar stapes and only a shallow pit where her oval window should have been. The facial nerve was dehiscent and lay across the oval window area. The round window niche was effaced and the round window was visible. The middle ear was mildly hypoplastic and the vertical portion of the facial nerve was in an abnormally anterior position, being easily visible when the tympanomeatal flap was elevated.

Analysis

The presence of a rudimentary stapes and absent oval window suggests a problem occurring in the seventh week. The facial nerve is expected to be low, perhaps overlying the oval window area as in Case 10, and possibly dehiscent. The vertical portion of the nerve should be more anterior and lateral than normal.

Surgical Findings

Surgery for the right ear was performed by the author in 1982. The middle ear was markedly hypoplastic. Only a rudimentary stapes was present, and there was no evidence of an oval window. The facial nerve was dehiscent on its inferior surface and lay across the area where the oval window should have been. The small middle ear was in a relatively anterior position, and the facial nerve appeared lower and more anteriorly placed in the surgical field than normal. The malleus and incus were mobile but mildly malformed. Hearing was reestablished by creating a small fenestra in the promontory just below the dehiscent facial nerve and using a prosthesis connected to the malleus handle. The vertical portion of the nerve ran anterior to the posterior wall of the external canal, so entry by routine tympanotomy placed the surgeon posterior to nerve.

Discussion

The facial nerve was found approximately in the position predicted by Fig. 35 in Chapter 2 and similar to that seen in Case 10, which had developmental arrest at the same time. With modern high resolution CT, the condition of the stapes and absence of the oval window could have been well visualized, allowing accurate prediction of facial nerve position prior to surgery.

CONCLUSION

A precise description of the developmental anatomy of the facial nerve and associated ear structures has been organized in a convenient table (Chapter 2, Table 2). Application of this knowledge to eleven patients with congenitally malformed ears over a period of six years has been helpful. Because of the high incidence of facial nerve dehiscence even in the normally developed ear, predictions of incomplete fallopian canal development are less helpful than predictions of location. It seems wise in all ear operations to assume a portion of the nerve is exposed until surgical observation proves otherwise. Predictions of facial nerve position can be made with reasonable accuracy when based on proper analysis of developmental anomalies of other ear structures.

In cases in which the facial nerve canal is not developed, it may be impossible to obtain accurate localization of the facial nerve radiographically prior to surgery. In these cases, a judgment based on understanding of embryology may be the surgeon's only guide to the position of the facial nerve. Considerably more experience is necessary to establish the reliability and validity of this approach with certainty. Moreover, extreme caution must always be exercised when operating on an ear with congenitally abnormal anatomy. However, it should not be necessary for the surgeon to approach the congenitally malformed ear with the fear that "you never know where the facial nerve is going to be." Otologic surgery can be planned accurately and carried out safely and expeditiously through comprehensive understanding and application of the embryology of the facial nerve and ear.

4

Isolated Anomalies of the Facial Nerve

A congenital anomaly of the ear, or the presence of a syndrome involving the ear or other body systems, alerts the surgeon to the possibility of anomalous facial nerve position. However, variations in facial nerve anatomy occur even in the absence of other abnormalities. Sometimes unusual facial nerve development can be identified preoperatively through radiologic imaging, but often it is not detected until the nerve is exposed surgically. Consequently, it is essential for the otologist to be aware of the many variations of facial nerve configuration that have been reported, and to be alert for them in every patient. Proctor and Nager (1, 2) published a particularly comprehensive review of normal and abnormal fallopian canal anatomy, and their articles are useful supplements to the material presented in this book.

Numerous facial nerve arrangements may be found in the temporal bone. Figure 1 illustrates some of the reported configurations. Such facial nerve variations may occur alone. However, the presence of ossicular anomalies (3–6) should make the surgeon particularly wary, including even minor anomalies, such as a malformed stapes, not identified until surgery.

DEHISCENCE OF THE FACIAL NERVE

Dehiscence of the fallopian canal is the most common "abnormality" encountered. In fact, it occurs so frequently that it is almost inappropriate to consider it abnormal. Its frequency is not surprising when one considers its complex development from two embryologic structures: Reichert's cartilage and the otic capsule. In fact, the portion contributed by Reichert's cartilage can be identified histologically until approximately the end of the first year of life when ossification of the fallopian canal is usually completed (2). Dehiscences occur most commonly in the horizontal portion of the fallopian canal above the oval window. However, a dehiscence may occur in any portion of the nerve. Defects in other portions of the nerve are more likely to occur over the lateral aspect of the geniculate ganglion, near the cochleariform process, or in the vertical portion, than over the superior aspect of the nerve or medial to the geniculate ganglion. They may be as small as 0.5 mm, or may expose the entire horizontal and labyrinthine segments (Fig. 1).

Dehiscence of the facial nerve in the horizontal portion may be associated with bulging of the facial nerve in the region of the oval window. In an otosclerotic ear, this is usually obvious as a white mass obscuring the footplate and pressing against the stapes crura. However, in a chronically diseased ear, especially in the presence of cholesteatoma, protruding nerve may be mistaken easily for disease and inadvertently biopsied. This will cause facial paralysis. Such complications can be avoided through wider exposure and identification of the facial nerve prior to manipulation in this particularly hazardous area.

The true incidence of dehiscence is uncertain. Politzer (7), Fowler (8), Guild (9), Cawthorne (10), Hough (3), Kaplan (11), and others recognized many years ago the occurrence of fallopian canal dehiscence, but their estimates of its incidence varied from 7% to over 50%. In 1962, Beddard and Saunders (12) reported examining 52 fresh cadaver temporal bones under 16 power magnification and finding a 25% incidence of dehiscence. All of the defects were located above the oval window. They averaged 2 × 3 mm, but in one case the facial nerve was exposed throughout its middle ear course. More accurate estimates are gleaned from histologic studies. In 1961, Dietzel (13) studied 211 temporal bones and reported an incidence of 57% dehiscence. The vast majority were located adjacent to the oval window. His findings were similar to the definitive work of Baxter (14) published in 1971. He examined 535 temporal

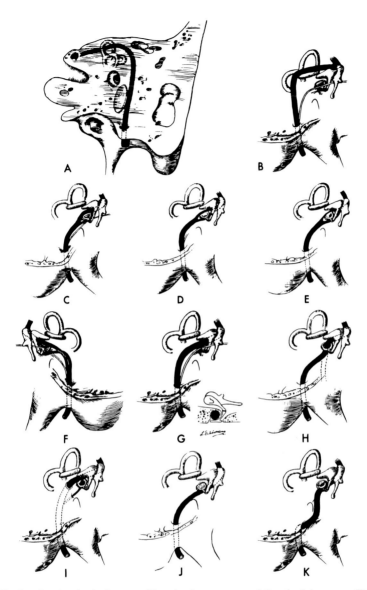

FIG. 1. Anatomical abnormalities in the course of the facial nerve. The facial nerve is seen bypassing the internal auditory canal and entering through the subarcuate fossa **(A)**, coursing along the superior aspect of the horizontal semicircular canal **(B)**, bifurcating proximal to the oval window **(C–F)**, coursing horizontally over the oval window **(G)**, coursing through the obturator foramen **(H,I)**, coursing between the oval window and round window **(J)**, coursing posteriorly inferior to the round window **(K)**. **FIG. 1.** *Continues.*

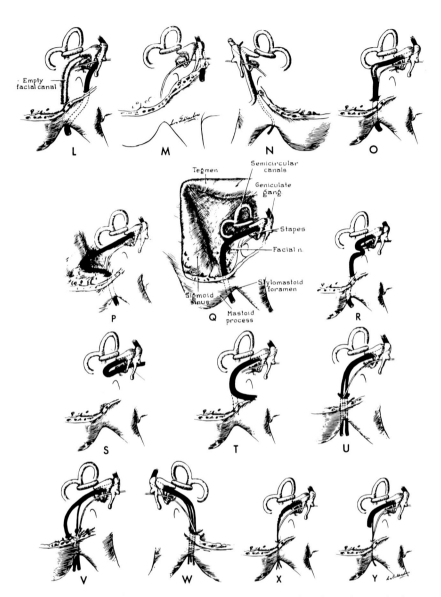

FIG. 1. *Continued.* The facial nerve is seen coursing from the geniculate ganglion straight downward over the promontory **(L)**, coursing through the anterior wall of the external auditory canal **(M)**, hypoplastic **(N,X,Y)** following an abnormal posterior, lateral, or anterior course through the mastoid **(O–T)**, and bifurcating or trifurcating distal to the oval window **(U–W)**. (From ref. 2, with permission.)

bones from the Massachusetts Eye and Ear Infirmary's collection and reported an incidence of 55% dehiscence. Ninety-one percent were located in the horizontal portion, and 9% were in the mastoid portion. Eighty-three percent of those in the tympanic segment were adjacent to the oval window and involved the lateral, inferior, and medial portions of the fallopian canals. The facial nerve protruded from its canal in 20%. Dehiscences ranged in diameter from 0.5 to 3.1 mm in most cases. In 0.8%, the dehiscence involved the entire tympanic segment. In some cases, this arrangement may be extremely hazardous (Fig. 2). Seventy-nine percent of mastoid dehiscences opened into the sinus tympani or into the retrofacial air cells. The size of mastoid dehiscence ranged from 0.4 to 2 mm, and the facial nerve protruded from the fallopian canal in 12% of cases. Because the incidence of dehiscence exceeds 50%, it is reasonable to consider it a normal variant rather than an anomaly. These studies did not investigate dehiscence of the facial nerve into the middle fossa. Intracranial exposure of the facial nerve through the hiatus of the middle fossa floor is also extremely common.

VARIATIONS IN POSITION OF THE FACIAL NERVE

In 1961, Fowler (15) reported seven variations in facial nerve position and angulation. As illustrated in Proctor's work summarized in Fig. 1, the otologist must assume that almost any configuration is possible. In a review of 500 temporal bones, Basek (16) found three in which the facial nerve bifurcated within the temporal bone. Bifurcation may occur as far proximal as the geniculate ganglion (4), and branches such as the chorda tympani may also bifurcate (17). It has even been suggested that motor fibers of the facial nerve may travel with the chorda tympani nerve, although this has not been well documented (18). Because of the multiplicity and complexity of facial nerve variations, it is convenient to consider them by anatomic region. Anomalies in the intracanalicular portion of the facial nerve are uncommon. The intracanalicular segment of the nerve is approximately 1 cm in length. Rarely, the facial nerve may bifurcate within the internal auditory canal (2). Even more rarely, it may enter the temporal bone through the subarcuate fossa

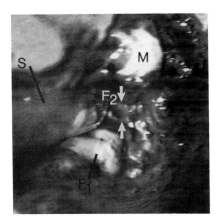

FIG. 2. Photograph of a facial nerve encountered during repair of a temporal bone fracture. A fragment of middle fossa floor had been displaced inferiorly and crushed the facial nerve, which was dehiscent throughout its entire tympanic (F_1) and labyrinthine (F_2 and *white arrows*) segments. A suction (S) and the malleus head (M) are also visible.

rather than through the internal auditory canal, coursing through the arch of the superior semicircular canal directly to the stylomastoid foramen (19). Bifurcation of the facial nerve in the labyrinthine segment is also rare (20, 21). The labyrinthine segment varies between 2.5 and 6 mm (22). It is important for the otologist, especially the neurotologist, to be familiar with anomalies in this region. For example, although entry of the facial nerve through the subarcuate fossa is rare, this anomaly puts the facial nerve at great risk during labyrinthectomy or translabyrinthine procedures.

Unusual facial nerve position in the tympanic segment is of most frequent interest to the otologist. Many of the potential anomalies are illustrated in Fig. 1. The tympanic segment varies in length from 7 to 11 mm (22). Bifurcations of the facial nerve anterior to the oval window have been observed on many occasions and are often associated with anomalies of the oval window and stapes (2). In one case, one portion of a bifid facial nerve passed through the obturator foramen of the stapes (23). Several other authors have reported a single (nonbifurcated) facial nerve coursing between the crura (20, 24, 25). Anomalous facial nerve placement inferior to the oval window has been reported in several patients with congenitally fixed stapes (26, 27). However, this anomalous position may occur in patients without congenital conductive hearing loss, as well (17, 28, 29). The facial nerve has also been reported coursing straight from the geniculate ganglion to outside the temporal bone (30), having an abnormally wide angle near the geniculate ganglion (31), coursing through the anterior wall of the external auditory canal (15), appearing hypoplastic (32), and with other abnormalities. Dickinson et al. (33) reported a facial nerve coursing across the promontory anterior to both the oval and round windows and exiting the temporal bone through the hypotympanum, associated with an empty facial canal in normal position. However, this unique report must be viewed with skepticism because all other evidence indicates that differentiation of the primordial otic capsule into a fallopian canal is initiated in response to contact with the nerve. There is no evidence that there is genetic information that would permit fallopian canal development in the nerve's absence; in all other reports of anomalous facial nerve position, the fallopian canal has followed the anomalous course of the nerve. Consequently, if a normal fallopian canal is identified radiographically, the surgeon may be reasonably confident that the facial nerve is contained within it. Naturally, bifurcated or trifurcated nerves may course in part outside the canal.

Numerous facial nerve anomalies may be found in the mastoid segment (Fig. 3). The mastoid segment varies in length between 9 and 16 mm (34). The nerve may exit the middle ear and enter the mastoid more anteriorly and cephalad than normal (35), course more posteriorly than usual adjacent to the sigmoid sinus (15, 36–38), and lesser posterior displacement may also occur with the nerve coursing 2 to 4 mm posterior to its usual location (39). The facial nerve may also course more anteriorly than normal (2), or may be S-shaped (40). One of the most frequent anomalies is a "dorsal hump" or bulge of the fallopian canal just distal to the horizontal semicircular canal (15, 38). This anomaly is particularly hazardous as it occurs in the portion of the facial nerve most commonly injured inadvertently during mastoid surgery. There have been numerous reports of facial nerve bifurcation and formation of separate fallopian canals (22, 41–43). The nerve may exit through individual stylomastoid foramina, or may reunite into a single trunk. Basek (16) reported a 0.6% incidence of bifurcation in 500 individuals.

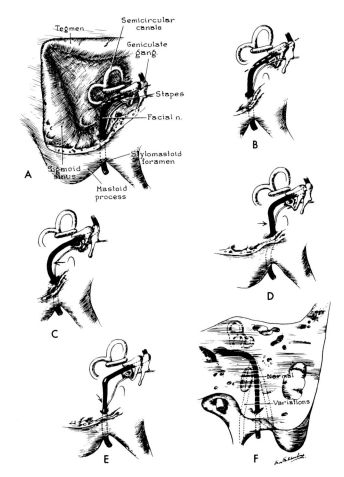

FIG. 3. Variations in the course of the facial nerve in the mastoid segment. The facial nerve is seen in normal position **(A)**, entering the middle ear of a slightly steeper angle than normal with the pyramidal bend slightly low **(B)**, following a slight anterior, posterior, or medial curve **(C–E)**, and following an outward oblique course **(F)**. An inward oblique course is rare. (From ref. 2, with permission.)

Trifurcation of the facial nerve with formation of separate canals has also been reported (44, 45). Dysplasia of the facial nerve has been observed as well (23, 43, 46, 47) and total agenesis may also occur, although it is usually associated with a syndrome such as thalidomide embryopathy (43) or Möbius' syndrome (48, 49) (see Chapter 5).

Variations also occur in the anatomy of the chorda tympani nerve. Ordinarily, the chorda tympani arises 5 mm proximal to the stylomastoid foramen (2). However, its origin may be anywhere from the geniculate ganglion to outside the stylomastoid foramen. External origin is uncommon, occurring in only 2% of cases (2). Rarely, the chorda tympani may join the facial nerve at the cochleariform process (13), and bifurcation of the chorda tympani nerve has also been seen (17). Abnormalities may also occur in the arteries and veins that accompany the facial nerve.

In addition, it has been suggested that there is a predilection for neuroma formation at the site of facial nerve dehiscence. Babin et al. (50) reported three such cases and suggested that they were traumatic neuromas caused by chronic inflammation with proliferation of neurofibrils. The possible relationship between fallopian canal dehiscence with facial nerve herniation and neuroma formation is also raised by Nager and Proctor (2), but such cases are exceedingly rare. There is no convincing evidence to establish a causal relationship or even tendency for association between the anomaly and neoplasm.

DISCUSSION

Numerous anomalies may occur in the course and relationships of the facial nerve, some of which were discussed in this chapter. Although the otologist expects abnormalities in the presence of congenital malformations of the ear, the surgeon may be less likely to anticipate them in an ear that appears normal. Careful attention must be paid to even minor anomalies such as small malformations of the external ear, preauricular cysts, unusual shape of the ossicular heads or stapes, or an abnormal radiologic study, as these may be suggestive of facial nerve abnormality. Conductive hearing loss in childhood should also raise the surgeon's suspicions. However, facial nerve anomalies occur even when all else is normal, so every patient undergoing otologic surgery must be approached with caution. It is advisable in all cases to identify normal structures such as the ossicles, round window, oval window, and cochleariform process, and to visualize the facial nerve and fallopian canal before manipulating the middle ear extensively. This is especially important in surgery for chronic otitis media, as the facial nerve may be surrounded by cholesteatoma or scar; its anomalous course will only be recognized prior to injury if the surgeon routinely establishes the course of the facial nerve early in every procedure.

REFERENCES

1. Proctor B, Nager GT. The facial canal: normal anatomy, variations and anomalies. *Ann Otol Rhinol Laryngol* 1982;91 (Suppl 93):49–60.
2. Nager GT, Proctor B. Anatomical variations and anomalies involving the facial canal. *Ann Otol Rhinol Laryngol* 1982;91 (Suppl 93):61–77.
3. Hough JVD. Malformations and anatomical variations seen in the middle ear during the operation for mobilization of the stapes. *Laryngoscope* 1958;68:1337–1379.
4. Caparosa RJ, Klassen K. Congenital anomalies of the stapes and facial nerve. *Arch Otolaryngol* 1966;83:420–421.
5. Sando I, English GM, Hemenway WG. Congenital anomalies of the facial nerve and stapes: a human temporal bone report. *Laryngoscope* 1968;78:315–323.
6. Hashimo T, Pararella MD. Middle ear anomalies. *Otolaryngol* 1971;94:235–239.
7. Politzer A. *A textbook of diseases of the ear and adjacent organs.* Philadelphia: Lea Brothers, 1894;450.
8. Fowler EP Jr, ed. *Medicine of the ear*, 2nd ed. New York: Thos. Nelson and Sons, 1947;121–122.
9. Guild SR. Natural absence of part of the bony wall of the facial canal. *Laryngoscope* 1949;59:668–673.
10. Cawthorne T. Membranous labyrinthectomy via the oval window for Meniere's disease. *J Laryngol Otol* 1957;71:524–527.
11. Kaplan J. Congenital dehiscence of the fallopian canal in middle ear surgery. *Arch Otolaryngol* 1960;72:197–200.
12. Beddard D, Saunders WH. Congenital defects in the fallopian canal. *Laryngoscope* 1962;72:112–115.
13. Dietzel K. Uber die dehiszen zen des facialiskanals. *Z Laryngol Rhinol Otol* 1961;40:366–374.
14. Baxter A. Dehiscence of the fallopian canal. *J Laryngol Otol* 1971;85:587–594.
15. Fowler EP Jr. Variations in the temporal bone course of the facial nerve. *Laryngoscope* 1961;71:937–946.
16. Basek M. Anomalies of the facial nerve in normal temporal bones. *Ann Otol Rhinol Laryngol* 1962;71:382–390.
17. Duncan DJ, Shea JJ, Sleeckx JP. Bifurcation of the facial nerve. *Arch Otolaryngol* 1967;86:619–631.
18. Gasser R, May M. Embryotic development of the facial nerve. In: May M, ed. *The facial nerve*. New York: Thieme, 1986;13.
19. Dworacek H. Die anatomisehen verhaltnisse des mittelohres unter operationsmieroscopischer betrachtung. *Acta Otolaryngol (Stockh)* 1960;51:31–45.

20. Altmann F. Zur anatomic und formalen genese der atresia auris congenita. *Monatsscher Ohrenheilkd Laryngo Rhino* 1933;67:765–771.
21. Miehlke A, Partsch CJ. Ohrmissbildung: facialis und aldueenslahmung als syndrom der thalidomidschadigung. *Arch Ohren Heilk Z Hals Heilk* 1963;181:154–174.
22. Arndt HJ. Zweiteilung des nervus facialis zwischen ganglion geniculi und foramen stylomastoideum. *HNO (Berlin)* 1967;15:116–118.
23. Marquet J. Congenital malformations and middle ear surgery. *J R Soc Med* 1981;74:119–128.
24. Butler GE. Transstapedial congenital malposition of the facial nerve. *Arch Otolaryngol* 1968;88:268.
25. Ombredanne M. Chirurgie des surdites congenitales par malformation ossiculaire. *Ann Otolaryngol (Paris)* 1960;77:423.
26. Martin H, Martin C. Anomaly of the facial nerve pathway and congenital ankylosis of the footplate. *J Fr Otorhinol Laryngol Chir Maxill-Fac* 1977;26:543–545.
27. Mayer TG, Crabtree JA. The facial nerve coursing inferior to the oval window. *Arch Otolaryngol* 1976;102:744–746.
28. Leek JF. An anomalous facial nerve: the otologist's albatross. *Laryngoscope* 1974;81:1535–1544.
29. Henner H. Congenital middle ear malformations. *Arch Otolaryngol* 1960; 17:154–158.
30. Sando I, Hemenway WG, Morgan WR. Histopathology of the temporal bone in mandibulofacial dysostosis (Treacher Collins syndrome). *Trans Am Acad Ophthalmol Otolaryngol* 1968;72:913–924.
31. Sando I, Leiberman A, Bergstrom L, et al. Temporal bone findings in Trisomy 18 syndrome. *Arch Otolaryngol* 1970;91:552–559.
32. Kodama A, Sando I, Meyers EN, Hashida Y. Severe middle ear anomaly with underdeveloped facial nerve. *Arch Otolaryngol* 1982;108:93–98.
33. Dickinson JT, Srisomboon P, Kamerer DB. Congenital anomaly of the facial nerve. *Arch Otolaryngol* 1968;88:357–359.
34. Kullman GL, Dyek PJ, Cody TR. Anatomy of the mastoid portion of the facial nerve. *Arch Otolaryngol* 1971;93:29–33.
35. Altmann F. Congenital atresia of the ear in man and animals. *Ann Otol Rhinol Laryngol* 1955;64:824–858.
36. Kettel K. *Peripheral facial palsy: pathology and surgery*. Springfield, Illinois: Charles C. Thomas, 1959;26.
37. Wright J Jr, Taylor C, McKay D. Variations in the course of the facial nerve as illustrated by tomography. *Laryngoscope* 1967;77:717–733.
38. Kettel K. Abnormal course of the facial nerve in the fallopian canal. *Arch Otolaryngol* 1946;44:406–408.
39. Kettel K. Surgery of the facial nerve. *Arch Otolaryngol* 1963;77:327–341.
40. Glasscock M. Unusual facial nerve problems. *Laryngoscope* 1971;91:669–683.
41. Hahlbrock K. Zweiteilung des N. facialis im Warzenfortsatz. *Arch Ohren usw Heilk u Z Hals-usw Heilk* 1960;174:465–469.
42. Wright JW. Polytomography and congenital external and middle ear anomalies. *Laryngoscope* 1981;91:1806–1811.
43. Miehlke A. *Surgery of the facial nerve*. Munich: Urban and Schwarzenberg Verlag, 1973. Philadelphia: WB Saunders, 1972.

44. Botman JW, Jongkees LBW. Endotemporal branching of the facial nerve. *Acta Otolaryngol (Stockh)* 1955;45:111–114.
45. Heermann J Jr. Zwei und dreigeteilter facialis in der pauke mit aplasie des ovalen fensters, facialis neurinom unter dem ambossehenkel. *Z Laryngol Rhinol* 1967;46:451–457.
46. Hawley CW. Abnormalities of the mastoid with special reference to the facial nerve. *Illinois Med J* 1922;41:116–120.
47. Tobeck A. Ueber den verlauf des facialiskanals im roentgenbild. *Arch Ohren Nasen Kehlkopfheilkd* 1938;144:276.
48. Altmann F. Problem of so-called congenital atresia of the ear. *Arch Otolaryngol* 1949;50:759–788.
49. Sando I, Ikeda M, Kitajiri M, May M. Histopathology of the facial nerve, temporal bone. In: May M, ed., *The facial nerve.* New York: Thieme, 1986;122–124.
50. Babin RW, Fratkin J, Harker LA. Traumatic neuromas of the facial nerve. *Arch Otolaryngol* 1981;107:55–58.

5

Structural, Congenital, and Hereditary Abnormalities

Abnormalities of the facial nerve may occur in conjunction with other malformations of the ear, in isolation without associated anomalies, or in conjunction with a variety of syndromes that include abnormalities elsewhere in the body. It is useful for the otologist to be familiar with the many syndromes that have been associated with facial nerve disorders. In this book, we shall consider only those syndromes associated with structural, congenital, and/or hereditary abnormalities. Facial paralysis may also be caused by a variety of acquired conditions such as Guillain-Barré syndrome, Ramsay Hunt syndrome (herpes zoster oticus), Bell's palsy, multiple sclerosis, Duchenne's syndrome, various infectious diseases, and other conditions. However, the differential diagnosis of acquired causes of facial paralysis is covered extensively in many other sources and will not be addressed here.

Congenital and hereditary facial paralysis warrant special mention. Although congenital facial paralysis should always make one consider a syndrome, birth trauma is probably a more common cause, especially in the absence of other congenital anomalies. A history of forceps delivery, prolonged labor, or findings of ecchymosis over the mastoid or of hemotympanum suggest birth trauma. The presence of bilateral facial paralysis, other cranial nerve deficits, or other anomalies suggest a developmental etiology. Early, accurate diagnosis is important if the etiology is traumatic. In some cases, surgery and facial nerve repair may be required in the newborn. If the cause is not traumatic, treatment is generally delayed except for eye protection.

Good reviews of the differential diagnosis of facial paralysis in newborns are available in the literature (1, 2). Most hereditary conditions that include the deformity of facial paralysis show it at the time of birth. However, a few hereditary syndromes are associated with the development of facial paralysis later in life. In addition, many hereditary and congenital malformations are associated with abnormal facial nerve anatomy in the presence of normal nerve function. It is important for the clinician to be familiar with these conditions because the abnormal position puts the nerve at increased risk of injury during surgery. In addition, many such problems are associated with malformations of the middle ear. So there is an increased likelihood that such patients will be exposed to the risks of ear surgery and possible facial nerve injury.

SYNDROMES ASSOCIATED WITH FACIAL NERVE ABNORMALITIES

Anencephaly

Anencephaly, a severe malformation of the head, represents a developmental defect of both the skull and brain resulting from failure of closure at the anterior portion of the neurogroove to form an intact neural tube. Secondary consequences of this profound malformation include altered facial structure and auricular development. The facial nerve course is frequently abnormal and may cross the petrous pyramid or the middle ear.

Altmann (3) described the postmortem ear examination of three anencephalic newborns. In two cases, the facial nerve and geniculate ganglion were normal in size. In the third case, they were slightly hypoplastic. The course of the facial nerve was normal, except on one side of one case.

Bogorad's Syndrome

The syndrome of lacrimation while eating was described in detail by Bogorad (4) in 1928, and he referred to it as the "syndrome of crocodile tears." In many reported cases, the syndrome has occurred subsequent to facial palsy. Ford (5) noted that this syndrome occurs only when the lesion is proximal to the geniculate ganglion. During regeneration, some fibers destined for the submandibular and sublingual glands may become rerouted to the lacrimal gland. Thus lacrimation occurs when gustatory stimuli are present. This syndrome has also been seen in association with neurosyphilis, which may be congenital, and following facial palsy of many other causes such as herpes zoster, which may also be acquired at birth (6).

Bulbopontine Paralysis with Progressive Sensorineural Hearing Loss

Bulbopontine paralysis with progressive sensorineural hearing loss is a syndrome characterized by autosomal recessive inheritance. It is seen more commonly in females (7). It is distinguished from juvenile amyotrophic lateral sclerosis by the impressive involvement of bulbar musculature and associated progressive bilateral sensorineural hearing loss, which may be the first symptom. The disease usually presents in childhood with a slowly progressive onset of bulbar palsy and facial weakness, dysphagia, and dysarthria. Often tongue fibrillations are observed. Although facial paresis is common, complete facial paralysis does not usually occur.

Congenital Heart Disease

Congenital anomalies of the temporal bone have been reported to occur with other congenital anomalies including congenital heart disease (8–10). Egami et al. (10) reported on 10 cases of temporal bone anomalies and associated congenital heart disease. This paper is noteworthy because the subjects ranged in age from 1 to 35, thereby providing particularly valuable information for the otologic surgeon. Their findings included multiple middle ear anomalies owing to developmental arrest. Mesenchymal tissue remnants were present, and a high jugular bulb and stapedial artery persistence were observed. The angle of the facial nerve in the region of the geniculate ganglion was obtuse, along with large horizontal fallopian canal dehiscence. Surgical advances in the treatment of congenital heart disease are so successful that some such patients are likely to undergo otologic surgery for hearing improvement. In the presence of congenital heart disease, middle ear anomalies and abnormal facial nerve position should be anticipated.

Cojoined Twins

The occurrence of cojoined twins is rare, occurring in 1 out of every 50,000 to 60,000 births, with thoracopagus being the most commonly reported type (11). Relevant reports on temporal bone findings in cojoined twins are scarce, although an interesting case was reported by Igarishi et al. (12) in 1974. They examined the temporal bones from a thoracopagus cojoined twin and found a malformed facial nerve on one side and an underdeveloped petrous bone with aplastic inner ear apparatus on the other side.

Deleted Chromosome Syndrome

Chromosome deletions usually produce profound malformations affecting multiple body systems. Bergstrom et al. (13) reported temporal bone findings in multiple infants with physical abnormalities attributed to deletion of chromosomal material in the D group. The abnormalities they observe included stapes malformations, cochleosaccular abnormalities, and facial nerve hypoplasia.

Diabetes

Diabetes mellitus is an extremely common heritable disease. An increased incidence of diabetes has been recognized in patients who present with facial paralysis (14–16). Depending on the study, the incidence ranges from 10 to 66%. This has led to the routine practice among neurotologists of screening all patients with facial palsy for the presence of diabetes mellitus. Some investigators believe that facial palsy in a diabetic is a mononeuropathy, although no mechanism has been proven. In fact, a causal relationship has not been established, and all one can say with certainty is that diabetes mellitus predisposes a patient to the development of facial paralysis. In general, the palsy recovers spontaneously and behaves like idiopathic facial paralysis (Bell's palsy) in nondiabetics.

DiGeorge Syndrome

This syndrome of multiple anomalies of craniofacial, cardiovascular, and visceral structures, along with absence or hypoplasia of the thymus and parathyroid glands, bears the name of the scientist who first described it (17). Few reports exist in the literature. However, based on varied clinical patterns observed in patients with DiGeorge syndrome, Lischner (18) further categorized the syndrome as follows: (a) III–IV pharyngeal pouch syndrome; (b) DiGeorge syndrome, thymic agenesis; and (c) partial DiGeorge syndrome, thymic hypoplasia.

The craniofacial and aural anomalies associated with this syndrome range from minimal to severe. Black et al. (19) report temporal bone findings in a patient with partial DiGeorge syndrome. The infant had severe symmetric malformations of the outer, middle, and inner ears. Owing to the massive developmental arrest of aural structures, it was inferred that this individual would have been deaf. The facial nerve was found to be hypoplastic with an abnormal course on one side. Although facial nerve function could not be evaluated in this infant with partial DiGeorge syndrome, facial paralysis has been reported in DiGeorge syndrome (20).

Dominant Craniometaphyseal Dysplasia

Craniometaphyseal dysplasia (CMD) was named by Jackson et al. (21) in 1954. The two major features of this hereditary bone disease are metaphyseal widening of the limbs and bony overgrowth of the facial bones and skull. Clinical findings are generally not prominent at birth, but they become evident in early infancy or childhood. Most researchers agree that the mode of inheritance is dominant transmission (22–24).

The otolaryngologic features of CMD include narrowed nasal passages and nasal dorsum deformity, obliteration of the paranasal sinuses and mastoid air cells, conductive and sensorineural hearing loss, and bony overgrowth of the facial bones. Unilateral and bilateral facial paralysis have been reported. Kietzer and Paparella (25) reported four patients with CMD in 1969. Each patient had many of the abnormalities described above. Two had unilateral facial paralysis. Disturbance of facial nerve function is thought to be secondary to bony encroachment of the facial nerve in the temporal bone.

Dystrophia Myotonica

An expressionless face is the predominant characteristic of dystrophia myotonica. This is a steadily progressive, familial distal myopathy that affects the muscles of the face, jaw, neck, and eyelids. Congenital facial diplegia appearing in association with this disease at birth is the severest form. Because the facial muscles, temporal, and masseter muscles are atrophic, the usual animation and innervation procedures are not helpful in treating these patients.

Hemifacial Microsomia

Hemifacial microsomia consists of unilateral microtia, macrostomia, and failure of the mandibular ramus and condyle to form. Most research has revealed no evidence that this disease is inherited (26). Walker (27) suggests that it is caused by a disturbance during intrauterine development, possibly in the 20 to 25 mm stage. Facial manifestations include striking facial asymmetry, which is partially owing to hypoplasia of the pinna. The maxillary and malar bones of the affected side are small and flattened. Ear malformations range from complete aplasia to a crumpled, distorted pinna. Often the ear canal is absent (27–30). Facial palsy has been reported (31, 32). Although the palate is usually normal, high asymmetric palatal arches have been reported (33), as have cleft lower lip (34) and parotid aplasia (35). Other findings may include lower palpebral fissure, microthalmia, strabismus, coloboma of the iris and choroid, congenital cystic eye, and pulmonary agenesis on the ipsilateral side.

Goldenhar's Syndrome

Goldenhar's syndrome is a rare group of anomalies representing defects in the morphogenesis of the first and second branchial arches, often accompanied by vertebral and/or ocular anomalies. Goldenhar's syndrome is distinguished from hemifacial microsomia by several factors as it includes epibulbar dermoids and/or lipodermoids, along with vertebral anomalies such as cervical fusion or spina bifida. It has been suggested by Weyers and Thier (36) that vertebral anomalies are more often associated with unilateral facial hypoplasia. This symptom complex also includes auricular appendices and pretragal blind-ended fistulas (37). This syndrome differs from hemifacial microsomia particularly in that its findings are bilateral. Goldenhar's syndrome occurs in 1 out of 5,000 births, affecting males more than females (38).

Hereditary Acoustic Neuromas

The syndrome of bilateral acoustic nerve tumors is transmitted through an autosomal dominant inheritance pattern. Symptoms are rarely apparent during infancy, usually appearing at approximately 20 years of age. Clinical manifestations result from tumor expansion and encroachment upon other cranial nerves. Sensorineural hearing loss is often the first sign. Other manifestations include palsies of the fifth, sixth, seventh, ninth, and tenth cranial nerves.

Melkersson-Rosenthal Syndrome

This is a rare disorder characterized by recurrent alternating facial paralysis. The cause is unknown, although Melkersson in his original writings described vasomotor instability and cerebral edema as causes of this phenomenon (39). Heredity may be a factor in Melkersson-Rosenthal syndrome since it has been observed in several members of the same family. The distinguishing features of this syndrome, in addition to the recurrent alternating facial palsy, include edema of the lips, face, and eyelids; cheilitis; and fissured tongue (40). Neurologic symptoms, in addition to the seventh nerve paralysis, include headache, blepharospasm, epiphora, hypogeusia, hyperhidrosis, and hearing loss (41–43).

Möbius' Syndrome

Möbius' syndrome is a rare congenital complex of anomalies including bilateral facial paralysis, unilateral or bilateral abducens paralysis, deformities of the extremities, aplasia of brachial and thoracic muscles, and often involvement of other cranial nerves. The lower four cranial nerves are involved most frequently, especially the hypoglossal. Heubner (44), Rainey and Fowler (45), and Spatz and Ulrich (46), as well as other investigators support Möbius' (47) theory of nuclear agenesis as the cause of this syndrome. Lennon (48) has suggested that nuclear atrophy occurs secondary to a mesodermal defect resulting in the failure of muscles to form.

The most prominent manifestations of this syndrome include a striking mask-like facies most apparent during laughing or crying, bilateral facial paralysis with the upper muscles of the face being more commonly involved, inability to abduct the eyes beyond the midline, and inability to close the eyes during blinking or sleeping. Ptosis is rare (49–51). However, epicanthus is common (49–52). Other abnormalities may include ear deformities, hearing loss, clubfoot, agenesis of digits, polydactyly, brachydactyly, and congenital dislocation of the hip. Often the lips, tongue, and larynx are paralyzed resulting in dysphonia (53). Saito et al. (54) described facial nerve findings in the temporal bone of a patient with Möbius' syndrome. Their extremely interesting report described the presence of a facial nerve that disappeared in the horizontal portion of the fallopian canal, thus supplying evidence that this syndrome may be caused by a peripheral lesion rather than a neural agenesis, in at least some cases.

Osteopetrosis Disease

Osteopetrosis, often referred to as "marble bone disease, " is an uncommon genetic disorder characterized by increased skeletal density. There are two forms of osteopetrosis: benign and malignant.

Benign osteopetrosis follows a dominant inheritance pattern. Most patients do not suffer frequent fractures, and many are totally asymptomatic. The diagnosis is often made incidentally following radiographic studies. Although facial paralysis is not routinely associated with benign dominant osteopetrosis, it occurs in some cases. When seen, it may be acute, recurrent, or progressive. In cases of recurrent facial paralysis, after several attacks the patient is frequently left with obviously reduced facial function. In one reported case, bilateral complete facial paralysis occurred (25).

Maglignant or autosomal recessive osteopetrosis is known as Albers-Schönberg disease. It involves a defect in the remodeling of bone and failure of absorption of the primary spongiosa. Clinical manifestations include neurological abnormalities from encroachment of bone on cranial nerves including facial paralysis, deafness, and blindness; anemia; hepatosplenomegaly; thrombocytopenia; and osteomyelitis. This disease may be recognized at birth. Death usually results in the first few years of life secondary to infection, and few patients survive to adulthood (55). Moderate mixed conductive and sensorineural hearing loss is seen in approximately 25 to 50% of patients (56, 57). Radiographic findings of the skull are very characteristic. The skull is thickened and dense. The mastoid bones are poorly pneumatized, as are the paranasal sinuses. The facial bones also appear more dense than normal. Temporal bone changes in one case study were described by Myers and Stool (57). They found a smaller than normal middle ear cavity with a portion of the facial nerve herniated into the middle ear. The fallopian canal was small and incomplete. Abnormal sclerotic bone was found throughout the temporal bone and the ossicles, as well. The stapes and round window were markedly thickened. There was no pneumatization of the mastoid cells. Acute and recurrent attacks of unilateral or bilateral facial paralysis occur, often beginning in the first few years of life. They are believed to be secondary to pressure from a dense bone on the intratemporal facial nerve.

Pierre Robin Syndrome

Pierre Robin syndrome consists primarily of micrognathia and glossoptosis secondary to hypoplasia of the mandible. A palatal cleft of varying degrees has been reported in over 50% of cases (58–60). The palatal deformities range from a high arched palate without cleft to a complete cleft of the hard and soft palate. Infants with this syndrome frequently experience episodes of cyanosis with difficulty swallowing and breathing, particularly because of their relative macroglossia.

The first complete report on temporal bone findings in this syndrome was written by Igarashi et al. (61) in 1976. They described multiple anomalies of the middle and inner ear as structural, as opposed to neural and end organ developmental anomalies. In their case report, the infant was found to have small facial nerves and a large bony dehiscence of the fallopian canal.

Recessive Craniometaphyseal Dysplasia

Recessive craniometaphyseal dysplasia is a congenital bone disease transmitted through an autosomal recessive inheritance pattern. The deformities seen with this disease are more severe then those seen in dominant craniometaphyseal dysplasia. The major features are glabella and paranasal prominence with severe mandibular prognathism. Nasal obstruction is generally complete with a resultant permanently opened mouth. Ocular hypertelorism is also characteristic. Progressive visual disturbance and blindness have been reported (62–64). Other otolaryngologic findings include unilateral facial paralysis and severe hearing loss, which is more often conductive than sensorineural.

Sclerosteosis

Sclerosteosis, an autosomal recessive syndrome, was probably first described by Hirsche (65) in 1929. This syndrome is characterized by generalized osteosclerosis, and hyperostosis of the mandible, calvarium, pelvis, and clavicles. Abnormalities of the digits also occur often, particularly syndactyly. Facial paralysis may be apparent at birth, but it often appears early in childhood. The paralysis is generally unilateral at first, but eventually it becomes bilateral (66). Hearing loss is a virtually constant feature of this syndrome. It is usually bilateral and may be conductive, sensorineural, or mixed. In addition to radiographs, which help confirm the diagnosis, serum alkaline phosphatase levels are markedly elevated (67).

Sickle-Cell Disease

Sickle-cell disease is a hemoglobinopathy seen primarily in blacks. There is no cure for the disease. It is characterized by recurrent attacks of fatigue, weakness, abdominal pain, anorexia, jaundice, and pallor caused by circulatory impairment from erythrocyte sickling. Both sensorineural hearing loss (68) and facial nerve paralysis (69) have been observed during sickle-cell crisis.

Thalidomide-Induced Malformations

It is well known that thalidomide use during the first trimester of pregnancy was responsible for a great number of congenital malformations. Typically, they include aplasia of the limbs; a flat hemangioma on the forehead, nose, and upper lip; congenital heart disease; and atresia of the esophagus, duodenum, or anus (70). External ear deformities are also common. Other aural anomalies include congenital labyrinthine aplasia, facial paralysis, and absence of the facial nerve (70–72).

Treacher Collins Syndrome

Treacher Collins syndrome is inherited as an autosomal dominant trait with variable expressivity. Miscarriage and early postnatal death are common (73). Otolaryngologic features of this syndrome include downward sloping palpebral fissures, malar hypoplasia, deformed pinnae, receding chin, fish-like mouth, and unusual projection of scalp hair that extends toward the lateral cheek. A high percentage of these patients also have lower lid coloboma and partial absence of the lower lid eyelashes (73). Both conductive and sensorineural hearing loss have been reported (74–76). Although facial paralysis is not a manifestation of this syndrome, several researchers have reported abnormal courses of the facial nerve on histopathologic examination, along with other multiple structural anomalies of the ear (77–80).

Trisomy 13 Syndrome

Trisomy 13 syndrome is associated with the presence of an extra chromosome in the D group of autosomes. The most common clinical manifestations of this syndrome include mental retardation; apneic spells; muscular hypertonia or hypotonia; eye defects; malformed ears; cleft lip and palate; polydactyly; multiple organ anomalies involving the heart, kidneys, testes, and uterus; hernias and hemangiomata of the skin (81). Common temporal bone findings are recognized through the report by Sando et al. (81) on 14 temporal bones. Facial nerve abnormalities include wide dehiscence of the fallopian canal, small facial nerve, and obtuse angle at the geniculate bend. In addition, ossicular abnormalities were common, and middle ear infections were seen in all cases.

Trisomy 18 Syndrome

Trisomy 18 syndrome is associated with an extra chromosome in the E group. The most common findings are low birth weight, mental retardation, hypertonicity, low set and/or malformed ears, prominent occiput, small mouth, micrognathia, high arched palate, congential heart disease, short sternum, hernia, limited hip adduction, flexion deformity of the fingers, finger and palm print abnormalities, renal anomalies, muscle hypoplasia, syndactyly of the second and third toes, and rocker-bottom feet (81). Reports of temporal bones findings in trisomy 18 syndrome are rare. Sando et al. (81) reported one case study in a female with this syndrome. Otologic findings included bilateral external auditory canal stenosis, multiple ossicular anomalies, incomplete fallopian canal, and abnormal courses of the facial and chorda tympani nerves. The facial nerve was underdeveloped, and the fallopian canal was dehiscent in several areas. The pyramidal eminence and stapedial tendon were absent, and the vertical portion of the facial nerve coursed more anteriorly than normal, traversing the middle ear anterior to a widely exposed stapedius muscles. The stapes was also malformed, and the facial nerve was in a position in which it could easily have been injured during surgery for hearing reconstruction.

Trisomy 21 Syndrome

Trisomy 21 (Down syndrome) was originally reported in 1866 (82). This syndrome has become one of the most widely recognized and described, partly because of its high incidence of one in every 660 births. Its most common features include hypotonia with open mouth and protruding tongue, small stature, awkward gait, mental retardation, brachycephaly with flat occiput, mild microcephaly, upslanting palpebral fissures, frontal sinus hypoplasia or aplasia, short hard palate, small nose with low bridge, epicanthal folds, Brushfield's spots of the iris, short neck, hand deformities, simian crease, foot deformities, pelvic malformations, cardiac anomalies in 40% of cases, and male hypogonadism.

The ears typically have small or absent ear lobes, small size, and often prominent and over-folding angulated upper helices. Igarashi et al. (83) provided one of the surprisingly few reports of temporal bone histology. Cochlear and vestibular abnormalities were present. Stapes malformation, pyramidal eminence underdevelopment, and stapedius muscle exposure into the middle ear were observed in one case. In one ear, an obtuse angle of the facial nerve was seen in the region of the geniculate ganglion. In one ear, an "exceptionally large vessel" coursed with the facial nerve. In all ears, the nerve itself and the geniculate ganglion were mildly hypoplastic, but no other pathology was observed.

Van Buchem's Disease

Van Buchem's disease, also known as hyperostosis corticalis generalisata, is a syndrome characterized by osteosclerosis of the skull, mandible, clavicles, and ribs; and hypoplasia of the diathyceal cortex of the long and short bones. The facial changes are not present at birth but usually become gradually apparent before the second decade. They include wide, thickened mandible reminiscent of acromegaly, although skull circumference is rarely enlarged. Mild exophthalmos may be present. The skull is thickened and the skull base becomes dense. Thickened clavicles become prominent. There is no increased incidence of fractures. Visual loss begins at approximately 30 years of age and progresses to optic atrophy and blindness. Of seven patients described by van der Wouden (84), all had bilateral symmetric hearing loss. Some were sensorineural, others were mixed. However, speech discrimination was reduced and tone decay was present in some cases.

Van Buchem described hearing loss in 13 of 15 patients, usually beginning at around 15 years of age (85). One patient was severely deaf by the age of 38. In the same report, two of 15 patients had unilateral facial paralysis, and one had bilateral facial paralysis. In a subsequent report of eight patients, all had facial paralysis (86). The facial palsy was bilateral in the five adults reported, and unilateral in the three children. Histologic sections of temporal bones have not been described, but autopsy examination has revealed narrowing of all cranial nerve foramina. Consequently, facial paralysis is believed to be owing to encroachment upon the nerve within the temporal bone. Additional findings include elevated alkaline phosphatase with normal serum calcium and inorganic phosphate levels.

Von Recklinghausen's Neurofibromatosis

The classic description of multiple skin tumors and cutaneous pigmentation was published by von Recklinghausen in 1882 (87). This syndrome of multiple neurofibromas is one of the three neurocutaneous syndromes that are associated with aural manifestations. The other two are Sturge-Weber syndrome and tuberous sclerosis. Von Recklinghausen's neurofibromatosis ordinarily follows an autosomal dominant inheritance pattern, although less than 50% of patients have an obvious family history of the disease. The incidence has been estimated at 1 in 2,000 in the general population, but it is much more common among patients with mental retardation (1 in 200) (88). The disease is characterized by multiple skin tumors, café-au-lait spots that appear within the first decade of 90% of patients, mental retardation in some cases, multiple eye anomalies, skeletal anomalies, and neurofibromas of various organs including the stomach, intestines, kidney, larynx, and heart. Although aural involvement is not common, neurofibromas may occur in the tongue, floor of mouth, or gingiva. Neurofibromas of the maxilla and mandible may also occur. Neuromas may involve all cranial nerves and may produce hearing loss and facial paralysis. Typically, neurofibromas grow to a large size before producing cranial nerve deficits. Facial paralysis may occur from neurofibromas of the facial nerve or adjacent structures. Facial palsy is also commonly seen after attempts at surgical removal of these tumors. Malignant degeneration has been estimated to occur in 3 to 12% of patients (89–90).

CONCLUSION

In addition to the conditions described in this chapter, there are undoubtedly many other congenital and hereditary conditions in which facial nerve abnormalities may occur. It is wise for the clinician to anticipate abnormal facial nerve anatomy whenever ear surgery is performed, but especially if even a minor congenital defect is observed. When facial paralysis occurs at birth, most physicians look agressively for a definable etiology. However, the same diligence is not always exercised in evaluating facial paralysis later in life. It is useful to constantly remember the existence of the many hereditary and nonhereditary systemic conditions that may produce facial paralysis during childhood or adult life, and other important causes of facial palsy including intracranial tumors, facial neuromas, parotid neoplasms, multiple sclerosis, and may other diseases. Attention to these important entities will prevent casual and injudicious diagnoses of "Bell's palsy, " and will help all otolaryngologists optimize medical and surgical care for our many patients with facial nerve pathology.

REFERENCES

1. May M, Fria TJ, Blumenthal F, et al. Facial paralysis in children: differential diagnosis. *Otolaryngol Head Neck Surg* 1981,89:841–848.
2. Harris JP, Davidson TM, May M, et al. Evaluation and treatment of congenital facial paralysis. *Arch Otolaryngol* 1983;109:145–151.
3. Altmann F. The ear in severe malformations of the head. *Arch Otolaryngol* 1957;66:7–25.
4. Bogorad FA. Symptoms of crocodile tears. *Vrach Delo* 1928;11:1328–1330.
5. Ford FR. Paroxysmal lacrimation during eating as sequela of facial palsy: syndrome of crocodile tears. *Arch Neurol Psychiatr* 1933,29:1279–1288.
6. Ford FR. Woodhall B. Phenomena due to misdirection of regenerating fibers of cranial, spinal and autonomic nerves: clinical observations. *Arch Surg* 1938;36:480–496.
7. Boudin G., Pepin B, Vernant JC, et al. Cas familial de paralysie bulbo-pontine chronique progressive avec surdite. *Rev Neurol (Paris)* 1971;124:90-92.
8. Konigsmark BW, Gorlin RJ. *Genetic and metabolic deafness*. Philadelphia: WB Saunders, 1976.
9. Adkins WY, Gussen R. Oval window absence, bony closure of round window, and inner ear anomaly. *Laryngoscope* 1974;84:1210–1224.
10. Egami T, Sando I, Myers E. Temporal bone anomalies associated with congenital heart disease. *Ann Otol* 1979:72–78.
11. Jenkins EW, Watson TR, Mosenthal WT. Surgery in cojoined twins. *Arch Surg* 1958;76:35–40.
12. Igarishi M, Singer DB, Alford BR, et al. Middle and inner ear anomalies in a conjoined twin. *Laryngoscope* 1974;84:1188–1201.
13. Bergstrom L, Hemenway WG, Sando I. Pathological changes in congenital deafness. *Laryngoscope* 1972;82:1777–1792.
14. Sherwin PJ, Thong MD. Bilateral facial nerve palsy: a case study and literature review. *J Otolaryngol* 1987;16:28–33.
15. Adour KK, Bell DN, Wingerd J. Bell's palsy: the dilemma of diabetes mellitus. *Arch Otol* 1974;99:114–117.
16. Adour KK, Wingerd J, Doty HE. Prevalence of concurrent diabetes mellitus and idiopathic facial paralysis. *Diabetes* 1975;24:449–451.
17. DiGeorge AM. In discussion of paper by Cooper MD, Peterson RDA, Good RA: a new concept of the cellular basis of immunology. *J Pediatr* 1965;67:907–908.
18. Lischner HW. DiGeorge syndrome(s). *J Pediatr* 1972;81:1042–1044.
19. Black FO, Spanier SS, Kohut RK. Aural abnormalities in partial DiGeorge syndrome. *Arch Otolaryngol* 1975;101:129–134.
20. Gatti RA, et al. DiGeorge syndrome associated with combined immunodeficiency. *J Pediatr* 1972;81:920–926.
21. Jackson WPU, Albright F, Drewry G, et al. Metaphyseal dysplasia, epiphyseal dysplasia, diaphyseal dysplasia and related conditions. *Arch Intern Med* 1954;94:871–885.
22. Gorlin R, Sedano HO. Craniometaphyseal dysostosis and grandiodiaphyseal dysostosis. *Mod Med* 1968;36:154–155.
23. Komins C. Familial metaphyseal dysplasia, (Pyle's disease). *Br J Radiol* 1954;27:560–675.

24. Mori PA, Holt JF. Cranial manifestations of familial metaphyseal dysplasia. *Radiology* 1956; 66:335–343.
25. Kietzer G, Paparella M. Otolaryngological disorders in craniometaphyseal dysplasia. *Laryngoscope* 1969;68:921–941.
26. May M. *The facial nerve*. New York: Thieme, 1986;408,470.
27. Walker DG. *Malformation of the face*. Edinburgh: Livingstone, 1961.
28. Braithwaite F, Watson J. A report on three unusually cleft lips. *Br J Plast Surg*, 1949;2:38–49.
29. Canton E. Arrest of development of the left perpendicular ramus of the lower jaw, combined with malformation of the external ear. *Tr Path Soc London* 1861;12:237–239.
30. Engel MB, Brodie AG. Condylar growth and mandibular deformities. *Surgery* 1947;22:976–992.
31. Ruchton MA. Malformation of the mandibular ramus treated by a bone graft. *Dent Rec* 1942;62:272–274.
32. Ogston A. On congenital malformation of the lower jaw. *Br J Dent Sc* 1875;-18:1–11,49–54,109–116.
33. Revazov BC. Intracerebral pathway of the facial nerve during human intra-uterine development. *Arkh Anat Gistol Embriol* 1958;35(5):106–107.
34. Halberg GP, Paunessa JM. An incomplete form of mandibulofacial dysostosis (Franceschetti's syndrome). *Br J Ophthalmol* 1949;33:709–713.
35. Entin MA. Reconstruction in congenital deformity of the temporomandibular complex. *Plast Reconstr Surg* 1958;21:461–469.
36. Weyers H, Thier CJ. Malformations mandibulo-faciales et dilimitation de'un syndome oculo-vertebral. *J Genet Hum* 1958;7:143–183.
37. Gorlin R, Pindborg J. *Syndromes of the head and neck*. New York: McGraw Hill, 1964;419–423.
38. Jones KL. *Smith's recognizable patterns of human malformations*. Philadelphia: WB Saunders, 1988;584.
39. Stevens H. Melkersson syndrome. *Neurology* 1965;15:263–265.
40. May M. *The facial nerve*. New York: Thieme, 1986; 187.
41. Broser F, Bender RM. Uber zentral-nerwose symptome ber cheilites granu-lomatosa miescher bzw. Melkersson-Rosenthal syndrome. *Newenarzt* 1958; 29:21–27.
42. Hornstein O. Uber die patthogenese des sogenannten Melkersson-Rosenthal syndromes. *Arch Kiln Exp Dermat* 1961;212:570–605.
43. Schuppener HJ. Zum Melkersson-Rosenthal syndrome. *Dtsch Gesundh Wes*, 1958;11:1598–1610.
44. Heubner O. Uber angeborenen Kernmangel (infantiler kunschwund Mobius). *Charite Ann* 1900;25:211–243.
45. Rainey H, Fowler JS. Congenital facial diplegia due to nuclear lesion. *Rev Neurol Psychiatr* 1903;1:149–155.
46. Spatz H, Ulrich O. Klinischer und anatomischer beltrag zu den angeborenen beweglichkeitsdefeckten im hirnnervenbereich. *Z Kinderheilk* 1931;51:579–597.
47. Mobius PJ. Uber infantilen kernschwund. *Munch Med Wchnschr* 1892;39:17–21,41–43,55–58.
48. Lennon MB. Congenital deficiency of muscle of the face and eyes. Reports of three cases. *California J Med* 1910;8:115–117.

49. Hellstrom B. Congenital facial diplegia. *Acta Paediatr* 1949;37:464–473.
50. Henderson JL. The congenital facial diplegia syndrome: clinical features, pathology and aetiology. *Brain* 1939;62:381–403.
51. Nisenson A, et al. Masklike facies with associated congenital anomalies (Möbius syndrome). *J Pediatr* 1955;46:255–261.
52. Van Buskirk C. Congenital facial diplegia. *U S Armed Forces Med J* 1951;2:1553–1555.
53. Evans PR. Nuclear agenesis, Möbius syndrome. The congenital facial diplegia syndrome. *Arch Dis Child* 1955;30:237–243.
54. Saito H, Kishimoto S, Furuta M. Temporal bone findings in a patient with Möbius syndrome. *Ann Otol* 1981;90:80–84.
55. Wong ML, Balkang TJ, Reeves J, et al. Head and neck manifestations of malignant osteopetrosis. *Otolaryngol Head Neck Surg* 1978;86:585–594.
56. Johnston CC, Lawy N, Ford T, et al. Osteopetrosis. A clinical, genetic, metabolic and morphologic study of the dominantly inherited benign form. *Medicine (Baltimore)* 1968;47:149–167.
57. Myers EN, Stool S. The temporal bone in osteopetrosis. *Arch Otolaryngol* 1969;89:460–469.
58. Douglas B. The treatment of micrognathia associated with obstruction. *Plast Reconstr Surg* 1946;1:300–308.
59. Weseman C. Congenital micrognathia. *Arch Otolaryngol* 1959;69:31–44.
60. Kishadden NS, Dietrich SR. Review of the treatment of micrognathia. *Plast Reconstr Surg* 1973;12:364–373.
61. Igarashi M, Filippone M, Alford BR. Temporal bone findings in Pierre Robin syndrome. *Laryngoscope* 1976;79:1679–1687.
62. Graf K. Die bedeutung des Pyle's syndrome (leontiasis ossea) fur die otorhino-laryngologie. *Z Laryngol Rhino Otol* 1965;44:438–445.
63. Jackson WPU, et al. Metaphyseal dysplasia, epiphyseal dysplasia, diaphyseal dysplasia and related constructions. *Arch Intern Med* 1954;94:871–885.
64. Sommer F. Erne besondere form eiver generalesierten hyperostose mit leontiasis ossea faciei et crana. *Radiol Clin* 1954;23:65–75.
65. Hirsche IS. Generalized osteitis fibrosis. *Radiology* 1929;13:44–84.
66. Konigsmark B, Gorlin R. *Genetic and metabolic deafness.* Philadelphia: WB Saunders, 1976;172–174.
67. Beighton P, Hameroma H, Dun L. The clinical features of sclerosteosis—a review of the manifestations in 25 affected individuals. *Ann Intern Med* 1976;84:393–397.
68. Konigsmark B, Gorlin R. *Genetic and metabolic deafness.* Philadelphia: WB Saunders, 1976;370.
69. May M. *The facial nerve.* New York: Thieme, 1986;402.
70. Jorgensen MB, Kristensen HK, Buch NH. Thalidomide-induced aplasia of the inner ear. *J Laryngol* 1954;78:1095–1101.
71. Lenz W, Knapp K. Die thalidomid-embryopathie. *Dtsch Med Wochenschr* 1962;87:1232–1242.
72. Miehlke A. Normal and anomalous anatomy of the facial nerve and an embryological study of the thalidomide catastrophe in Germany. *Trans Am Acad Ophthal Otol* 1963;1030–1044.
73. Konigsmark B, Gorlin R. *Genetic and metabolic deafness.* Philadelphia: WB Saunders, 1976;210–211.

74. Stovin JJ, Lyons JA, Clemens RL. Mandibulofacial dysostosis. *Radiology* 1960;74:225–231.

75. Kittel G, Fleischer-Peters A. Das ohr bei dysostose syndromen des schadels. *Z Laryngol Rhinol Otol*, 1963;42:384–397.

76. Partsch CJ, Hulse M. Verschieden schwerhorigkeitsfor men innerhabl einer francesschetti-familie. *Laryngol Rhinol* 1975;54:385–388.

77. Sando I, Hemenway WG, Morgan WR. Histopathology of the temporal bone in mandibulofacial dysostosis (Treacher Collins syndrome). *Trans Am Acad Ophthalmol Otolaryngol* 1968;72:913–924.

78. Altmann F. Congenital atresia of ear in man and animals. *Ann Otol* 1955;64:824–858.

79. Herberts G. Otological observations on the "Treacher Collins syndrome." *Acta Otolaryngol* 1962;54:457–465.

80. Livingston G. The establishment of sound conduction in congenital deformities of the external ear. *J Laryngol* 1959;73:231–241.

81. Sando I, Leiberman A, Bergstrom L, et al. Temporal bone findings in trisomy 18 syndrome. *Arch Otolaryngol* 1970;91:552–559.

82. Down JLH. Observations on an ethnic classification of idiots. *Clinical Lecture Reports London Hospital* 1866;3:259.

83. Igarashi J, Takahaski M, Alford BR, et al. Inner ear morphology in Down's syndrome. *Acta Otol* 1977;83:175–181.

84. van der Wouden A. Deafness caused by hyperostosis corticalis generalisata. *Pract Otorhinolaryngol* 1968;30:91–92.

85. van Buchem FS, Hadders NH, Hansen JF, et al. Hyperostosis corticalis generalisata. *Am J Med* 1962;33:387–397.

86. van Buchem FS. Hyperostosis corticalis generalisata. *Acta Med Scand* 1971;189:257–267.

87. von Recklinghausen F. *Ueber die multiplean firbroma der haut und ihre beziehung u den multiplen neuromen.* Berlin: A Hirschwald, 1882.

88. Borberg A. Clinical and genetic investigations into tuberous sclerosis and Recklinghausen's neurofibromatosis. *Acta Psychiatr Neurol* 1951;71 (suppl):11–239.

89. Holt JF, Wright EM. The radiologic features of neurofibromatosis. *Radiology* 1948;51:647–663.

90. Hosoi K. Multiple neurofibromatosis (von Recklinghausen's disease): with special reference to malignant transformation. *Arch Surg* 1931;22:258–281.

Subject Index

Subject Index

A

Acoustic ganglion, 37
Acoustic nerve, 31, 40, 42
  MRI, 82
Acoustic neuroma, hereditary,
  135
Afferent taste fibers,
  embryology, 30
Age, fetal, 19
  at developmental arrest, 91
  estimation criteria, 4–5
  see also Facial nerve,
    embryology; Ear,
    embryology
Albers-Schönberg disease,
  137
Ampullae, semicircular canal,
  76
Amyotrophic lateral sclerosis,
  131
Anencephaly, 130
Annulus, tympanic
  membrane, 79
Antrum, 85, 87
Aqueduct, cochlea, 80
Atresia
  external auditory canal,
    109–111

plate, 105, 106, 109–111
  in place of tympanic
    membrane, 94–97
Attic, 65
Auditory meatus (canal)
  external, 48, 51, 58, 59,
    65, 72, 75, 84
  absence, congenital, 91,
    92, 94, 106–108
  atresia, 109–111
  bilateral stenosis,
    101–106
  complete atresia,
    bilateral, 98–100
  congenital absence,
    106–108
  CT scan, 104
  left, defect, 95–97
  left, stenosis, 100–101
  narrow, 114–115
  ossicular mass, 99
  right defect, 95–98
  internal, 63, 66, 73, 78, 79,
    81, 82, 92
  ossification, 87
Auditory vesicle, 45
Auricle, 45–47, 57, 58, 70,
  84–85, 87